You don't have to

**USE THE FINGERTIP
LOW CALORIE GUIDE**

CHAPTER 15

to find out which foods are
200-350 calories
100-200 calories
50-100 calories
20-50 calories
20 calories or less

You'll find delicious surprises like these...

Under 20 calories:
1 dill pickle
1 cup spinach

Under 50 calories:
1 egg roll
1 cup popcorn

Under 100 calories:
1 extra light beer
4 ounces gefilte fish

Under 200 calories:
7 ounces beef stew with biscuits
7½ ounces macaroni and cheese

Under 350 calories:
13 ounces eggplant parmigiana
8 ounces oysters

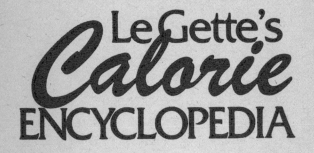

Le Gette's *Calorie* ENCYCLOPEDIA

Bernard Le Gette

WARNER BOOKS

A Warner Communications Company

WARNER BOOKS EDITION

Cover photo by Frank Marchesano

Warner Books, Inc.
666 Fifth Avenue
New York, N.Y. 10103

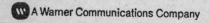 A Warner Communications Company

Printed in the United States of America

First Printing: January, 1983

10   9   8   7

Contents

v

Contents

Introduction

Losing weight is simple. It's not easy—but it's simple.
You cut the intake of your calories, and then
you lose weight. Everything else you've ever heard
is icing on the cake you can't eat. Carbohydrates,
cholesterol, volume, protein, metabolism, exercise,
are all very interesting, and confusing, to think
about, though none of these things plays a big role
in how much you weigh or how little you can
weigh.

But even when people cut calories they
usually don't do a very good job of it. You have
probably gone on diets, wondered why they
didn't work and wandered off them again, or maybe
they did work, but your will power collapsed—

the constant pressure of not eating so many delicious foods caved you right in.

There are two reasons why most people fail. The first is that they don't really know how many calories they're consuming. They estimate how many calories are in each food, estimate how much of each food they ate, and constantly say things like, "That was only a little snack—two or three crackers." Sound familiar? And of course they're always rejecting potatoes.

Well I'll tell you right now, there is no way you can estimate. You can't estimate the size, you can't estimate the number of calories and you can't estimate the number of times you snacked. You can't estimate a thing. You aren't that smart. Nobody is.

You have to count the pieces, weigh them, and check every time how many calories you just ate. And then you have to write it down. Every calorie. Every day.

Now I know this is more inconvenient than being fat, and hating yourself every day, and being tired, and having heart attacks. But that's the way it is. It does have the advantage of being one inconvenience instead of many, and it is also only one simple way to lose weight—instead of many complicated ways not to—which brings us to the second reason most people fail.

It's because losing weight tends to get very vague in people's minds. It's a hidden enemy

that has to be strained against every day. And that's
very disheartening—which means it won't work.
Any constant general restriction on your life, that
has no definite limits and no clear procedure,
is just not going to work. That's why specific diets
are so successful in the short term—they remove
the vagueness, the guesswork, the doubt. But we
aren't talking about the short term. We're talking
about weighing whatever you like for the rest of
your life.

Fortunately, you don't have to fight hidden
enemies. You don't even have to use much will
power. You only have to know how to count—
calories.

The purpose of this book and the years of
research that went into it is to give you—in
one place—the calories of all the foods you might
ever eat. Whether it's fresh, or a commercially
packaged brand, or a meal you ate in a restaurant
or prepared at home, or a snack you ate at a
drive-in—it's here. The portions listed are as
standardized as is practical, so you don't have
to bring your calculator. There are no extra columns
of things that won't help you lose weight, and
there is as little repetition as possible. You won't find
listings of Thingamajigs—25 calories; Thingamajigs
on a stick—25 calories; Thingamajigs sliced—25
calories, and so on. If thingamajigs are 25 calories,
that's all you need to read—very simple.

The chapters are in a logical order chosen to

LE GETTE'S CALORIE ENCYCLOPEDIA

help you remember where things are listed. If everything were listed alphabetically you wouldn't know if some fish would be found under fillet, or haddock, or Mrs. Paul's, and even when you found it you couldn't compare it to others of its kind. So everything is in these fourteen basic groupings.

And the fifteenth chapter is the Fingertip Low Calorie Guide. This is an innovation which I hope will enable you to find a variety of low calorie foods at a glance. They are listed in calorie groups so you can plan your shopping, your meals, even your snacks with a specific number of calories in mind. It is also a pretty thorough list of the low calorie foods available. As you'll see in the rest of the book, being called *low calorie* or *dietetic* is no guarantee that a food is low in calories.

Everything is listed for normal usage. That is, if a food is made from a mix, say, the quantity and the calories listed are for the food after it's been prepared according to the package instructions. Likewise, it is of no use to know how many calories are in a pound of spinach while it is still frozen, so that is not listed. Now some things are listed as containing 0 calories for one tsp, and that is accurate; it is also reasonably accurate for one tbs. I can't guarantee, however, that there are no calories in three lbs. of sweetener. There just might be a few.

So how do you lose weight? Eat *what* you want, though of course a balanced diet is always best. It's not what, but *how many* that counts. Remember, virtually all foods have calories. The question is, how much satisfaction and/or nutrition are you getting from a particular food? For the calories in it, a plain potato contains a phenomenal variety of nutrients— you can probably live longer on potatoes than on any other single food—and that would suit some people fine. Others, however, would like to go quickly on apples, which contain neither calories nor nutrients in any marked degree.

But however you do it—eat fewer calories. Measure every portion. It's quite easy. Just put your chicken, or your potato, on a scale, see what the scale says, and compare that to the portion listed in this book. Write down the number of calories for each meal. Add them up at the end of the day, and in the morning write down how much you weigh next to yesterday's calorie total.

But you have to do it every time. It won't do you any good sometimes. And if after awhile you think you can remember most foods' calories, you're wrong. You have to measure. You have to count. The reason you're fat (which is why you bought this book) is you don't know how to play it by eye. You were brought up to eat too much, your aggression makes you hungry, your metabolism is rotten, whatever. It doesn't matter. You want to be thin. I just told you how. If you really *want* to be thin, that's what you'll do. Otherwise you'll continue to play at it and make excuses.

Now if you want to look good and be completely healthy *in addition* to being thin, you'll also exercise, though the exercise won't do either of those things for you if you're overweight. And it won't help you to lose much weight either. The relation between calories and exercise is straightforward. The harder it is, the more calories you burn. There are 3,600 calories in 1 pound of fat. Roughly, you'll burn 100 calories by:

skating (either kind)	45	minutes
skiing (either kind)	35	"
football	30	"
handball	22	"
walking	19	"
rowing	18	"
bicycling	15	"
chopping wood	13	"
swimming	12	"
jumping rope	11	"
jogging	10	"
running	6	"

or (even more roughly) 18 holes of golf (on foot) or two sets of tennis.

So if you want to lose that pound of fat, it's easier not to eat the 3,600 calories than to jump rope for 7 hours. What will help the most is a regular, steady approach to food and calories. This book can be your guide to help you look and feel the person you really want to be.

1 quart	=	4 cups
1 cup	=	8 fluid ounces (oz)
1 cup	=	½ pint
1 cup	=	16 tablespoons
1 ounce	=	2 tablespoons
1 tablespoon (tbs.)	=	3 teaspoons
1 jigger, or shot	=	1½ ounces
1 pound (lb.)	=	16 ounces

Remember, a fluid ounce is a measure of volume, not weight.

ALL listings are for food *as prepared* for normal usage. That means that after it's been prepared with all the normal ingredients, and it's ready to eat—that's what the calories are for.

CHAPTER 1

Beverages

SPIRITS, WINES, LIQUEURS, COCKTAILS, BRANDIES, AND COCKTAIL MIXES

Note: The number of calories in distilled spirits depends entirely on the alcoholic content—the higher the proof, the higher the calories. This is true for bourbon, gin, rum, Scotch, tequila, vodka, and almost anything called whiskey.

1

Distilled Spirits, 1 oz

80 proof	65
90 proof	75
100 proof	85
150 proof	125

Cocktails, canned or bottled, alcoholic, 1 oz

Amaretto Sour
Mr. Boston   40
Apricot Sour
Party Tyme   33
Banana Daiquiri
Party Tyme   33
Daiquiri
Hiram Walker   59
Mr. Boston   33
Party Tyme   33
Calvert   63
Gimlet
Party Tyme   40
Gin & Tonic
Party Tyme   28
Mai Tai
Lemon Hart   60
Mr. Boston   36
Party Tyme   33

Manhattan
Calvert 54
Mr. Boston 40
Party Tyme 37

Margarita
Calvert 59
Mr. Boston 35
Mr. Boston strawberry 45
Party Tyme 33

Martini, Gin
Calvert 63
Hiram Walker 55
Mr. Boston 33
Party Tyme 41

Martini, Vodka
Calvert 63
Hiram Walker 49
Mr. Boston 34
Party Tyme 36

Old Fashioned
Hiram Walker 55

Piña Colada
Mr. Boston 60
Party Tyme 32

Rum & Cola
Party Tyme 28

Screwdriver
Mr. Boston 39
Party Tyme 35

1

Sour, Gin
Calvert 65
Sour, Scotch
Party Tyme 33
Sour, Tequila
Calvert 65
Sour, Whiskey
Calvert 60
Hiram Walker 60
Mr. Boston 40
Tequila Sunrise
Mr. Boston 40
Tom Collins
Calvert 65
Party Tyme 29
Vodka Tonic
Party Tyme 27
Wallbanger
Mr. Boston 34

Cocktail Mixes, bottled and dry, nonalcoholic, 1 oz or 1 premeasured packet

Alexander
Holland House 69
Amaretto
Holland House 79
Banana Daiquiri
Holland House 66

Beverages

1

Mint Julep
Holland House   67

Old Fashioned
Holland House   9
Party Tyme   28

Piña Colada
Holland House   60
Party Tyme   50

Pink Squirrel
Holland House   69

Planter's Punch
Party Tyme   37

Screwdriver
Holland House   69
Party Tyme   21

Sidecar
Holland House   17

Sour, Blackberry
Holland House   50

Sour, Virgin
Party Tyme   50

Sour, Whiskey
Canada Dry   11
Holland House   53
Holland House low calorie   9
Party Tyme   29
Party Tyme instant   53

Sip 'n Slim
Holland House   10

Strawberry Sting	
Holland House	35
Tom Collins	
Holland House	58
Party Tyme	44
Party Tyme instant	58

Cocktails, standard recipe, alcoholic, 1 oz alcohol, unless noted

Bacardi	155
Bloody Mary	140
Brandy Alexander	225
Bourbon Highball (1½ oz bourbon)	
with soda	125
with ginger ale	180
Cuba Libre	224
Daiquiri	135
Gimlet	136
Gin Fizz	172
Grasshopper	235
Irish Coffee	214
Manhattan	177
Martini, Gin or Vodka	115
Mint Julep	209
Old Fashioned	144
Orange Blossom	153
Pink Lady	190
Rob Roy	199

Rum Cola (see Cuba Libre)	224
Screwdriver	168
Side Car	161
Sloe Gin Fizz	155
Stinger	149
Tom Collins	170
Whiskey Sour	142

Wines, 4 oz

Alsatian
Wilm	88

Altar, red
Gold Seal	132
Henri Marchant	132

Blackberry
Manischewitz	180

Bordeaux
red
B&G Margaux	83
B&G Prince Noir	81
B&G Saint-Emilion	84
Chanson	108
Cruse	92
Cruse Saint-Emilion	92
Cruse Saint-Julien	92
Cruse Médoc	96
Cruse Château La Garde	108

Cruse Château Olivier — 108

white

B&G Graves — 87

Cruse Graves — 92

Burgundy

red

B&G Beaujolais St. Louis — 80

B&G Nuits St. George — 93

B&G Pommard — 89

Chanson Beaune — 108

Chanson Pommard — 108

Cruse Beaujolais — 96

Cruse Pommard — 96

Cruse Gevrey-Chambertin — 96

Gallo — 67

Gold Seal — 86

Henri Marchant — 84

Italian Swiss Colony — 86

Manischewitz — 85

Taylor — 99

sparkling

B&G — 92

Chanson — 96

Gold Seal — 97

Great Western — 109

Henri Marchant — 97

Lejon — 89

Taylor — 104

white

B&G — 83

Great Western	121
Taylor	120
Concord	
Gold Seal	132
Henri Marchant	132
Manischewitz	
red	160
white	130
medium dry	120
dry	85
Mogen David	160
Kosher	
Manischewitz	
sweet	170
medium	112
dry	91
Labrusca	
Gold Seal	130
Henri Marchant	132
Lake Country	
Taylor	106
Liebfraumilch	
Anheuser & Fehrs	80
Dienhard	95
Malaga	
Manischewitz	180
Moselle	
Dienhard	95
Julius Kayser	77

Great Western	96
Pinot Chardonnay	
Gold Seal	85
Henri Marchant	85
Louis Martini	120
Pinot Noir	
Inglenook	77
Louis Martini	120
Pouilly-Fumé	
B&G	80
Rhine	
Gold Seal	91
Dienhard	80
Gallo	67
Gallo Rhine Garten	78
Great Western	97
Henri Marchant	92
Julius Kayser	74
Inglenook	100
Italian Swiss Colony	86
Louis Martini	120
Taylor	92
Rhineskeller	
Italian Swiss Colony	88
Rice Wine	
Chinese	152
Japanese	286
Rhone	
Chanson	112

    B&G   93

Riesling

    Dienhard   96
    Gold Seal   92
    Henri Marchant   92
    Inglenook   82
    Louis Martini   120

Rosé

    Cruse   96
    Gold Seal   99
    Henri Marchant   96
    Italian Swiss Colony   86
    Taylor   92

Sake   151

Sancerre

    B&G   80

Sauterne

    Gallo   67
    Gallo Haut   83
    Gold Seal   97
    Gold Seal Haut   109
    Great Western   105
    Henri Marchant   109
    Italian Swiss Colony   77
    Louis Martini   120
    Mogen David cream   59
    Mogen David dry   39
    Taylor   105

Soave

    Antinori   110

Thunderbird
Gallo   139
Valpolicella
Antinori   109
Zinfandel
Inglenook   76
Italian Swiss Colony   80
Louis Martini   120

Aperitif and Dessert Wines, 4 oz

Asti Spumante
Gancia   168
Aquavit
Leroux   300
Campari   66
Dubonnet Blonde   151
Dubonnet Red   190
Madeira
Gold Seal   144
Henri Marchant   144
Leacock   160
Sandeman   168
Muscatel
Gallo   144
Gold Seal   210
Pernod
Julius Wyle   315

1

Port

Gallo	146
Gold Seal	185
Great Western	178
Italian Swiss Colony	170
Louis Martini	215
Robertson	180
Sandeman	184
Taylor	195

Sherry

Gallo	104
Gold Seal	185
Great Western	156
Taylor	200
Dry Sack	160

Sherry, cream

Gallo	150
Gold Seal	205
Great Western	180
Louis Martini	175
Taylor	178

Sherry, dry

Gallo	110
Gold Seal	162
Great Western	140
Italian Swiss Colony	132
Louis Martini	180
Sandeman	145
Taylor	152

Vermouth, dry

C&P	148
Gallo	100
Gancia	168
Great Western	113
Lejon	129
Noilly Pratt	136
Taylor	136

Vermouth, sweet

C&P	156
Gallo	150
Gancia	185
Great Western	172
Lejon	174
Noilly Pratt	172
Taylor	175

Cordials and Liqueurs, 1 oz

Amaretto	80
Anise	82
Anisette	
Bols	111
DuBouchett	85
DeKuyper	95
Garnier	82
Mr. Boston	90
Mr. Boston Connoisseur	64

Apricot

Bols	96
Dolfi	100
DuBouchett	65

B & B	94
Benai	110
Benedictine	110

Blackberry

Bols	90
Dolfi	89
DuBouchett	68

Brandy, flavored

Bols	100
DuBouchett	87
Garnier	6
Leroux	90
Mr. Boston	100
Mr. Boston Connoisseur	75

Cherry liqueur

Bols	96
DeKuyper	75
Dolfi	87
DuBouchett	72
Hiram Walker	82
Leroux	82

Chocolate

Vandermint	90

Claristine

Leroux	114

Coffee
Tia Maria	92
Pasha	100

Crème de almond
DuBouchett	100

Crème de apricot
Mr. Boston	90
Mr. Boston Connoisseur	65

Crème de banana
Garnier	90
Mr. Boston	90
Mr. Boston Connoisseur	65

Crème de cacao
Bols	100
Dolfi	100
DuBouchett	100
Garnier	100
Hiram Walker	100
Mr. Boston	90
Mr. Boston Connoisseur	65

Crème de cassis
Leroux	87
Mr. Boston	90

Crème de menthe 100
Crème de noisette 90
Crème de noyaux
Bols	115
Mr. Boston	99

Crème de peach
Mr. Boston Connoisseur	65

Curaçao	100
Drambuie	110
Grenadine	81
Kirsch	80
Kümmel	
DuBouchett	
48 proof	65
70 proof	83
Garnier	75
Hiram Walker	71
Leroux	75
Mr. Boston	78
Lochon Ora	
Leroux	89
Peach Liqueur	
Bols	96
DeKuyper	82
Dolfi	103
DuBouchett	67
Hiram Walker	81
Leroux	85
Raspberry Liqueur	
Dolfi	80
DuBouchett	56
Rock & Rye	
DuBouchett	
60 proof	78
70 proof	86
Garnier	83
Mr. Boston	90

Mr. Boston Connoisseur   65

Schnapps, peppermint
DuBouchett	85
Garnier	83
Hiram Walker	78
Leroux	87
Mr. Boston	77

Sloe Gin
Bols	85
DeKuyper	70
Dolfi	114
DuBouchett	70
Garnier	83
Mr. Boston	67

Triple Sec
Bols	104
Dolfi	107
DuBouchett	61
Garnier	83
Hiram Walker	105
Leroux	104
Mr. Boston	100

BEER, ALE, MALT LIQUOR,
12 oz

Andeker	160
Black Horse Ale	162
Brauhaus	150

1

Buckeye	144
Budweiser	156
Budweiser Malt Liquor	160
Busch Bavarian	155
Carling Black Label	160
Carlsberg Light	159
Carlsberg Dark	240
Champale Malt Liquor	157
Country Club Malt Liquor	163
Coors	138
Eastside Lager	145
Falstaff	150
Gablinger's	99
Goebel	145
Grand Union	150
Grenzquell	150
Hamms	138
Heidelberg	133
Heidelberg Light	129
Heileman's	158
Kingsbury	146
Knickerbocker	160
Meister Brau	144
Meister Brau Draft	144
Meister Brau Lite	96
Michelob	160
Michelob Light	134
Miller	150
Miller Lite	96
Natural Light	110

Old Dutch	150
Old Milwaukee	144
Old Ranger	150
Pabst Blue Ribbon	150
Pabst Light	100
Pabst Extra Light	70
Pearl	145
Pilser's	152
Red Cap Ale	159
Rheingold	160
Schaefer	158
Schlitz	148
Schlitz Light	96
Schmidt's	142
Stag	151
Stroh Bohemian	136
Stroh Bock	155
Stroh Light	115
Tuborg USA	140
Tudor	150

Near Beer, 12 oz

Goetz Pale	78
Kingsbury	45

1

Nonalcoholic Beer, 12 oz

Maltcrest	70
Metbrew	70
Zing	65

SOFT DRINKS, 8 oz

Note: Virtually all sodas that are called *low calorie*, *sugar free*, or *dietetic* contain 2 calories or less.

Aspen	105
Birch Beer	
Canada Dry	110
Pennsylvania Dutch	109
Yukon Club	116
Bitter lemon	
Canada Dry	104
Schweppes	128
Bitter orange	
Schweppes	124
Bubble Up	97
Cactus Cooler	120
Cherry	
Cott	123
Crush	121

Fanta	117
Mission	122
Club soda, all brands	0
Coconut	
Yoo-Hoo	117
Coffee	
Hoffman	88
Cola	
Canada Dry	110
Coca-Cola	96
Pepsi-Cola	104
Royal Crown	109
Pepsi Light	47
Shasta	90
Cream	
Canada Dry	127
Fanta	130
Shasta	90
Schweppes	115
Dr. Brown's Cel-Ray Tonic	89
Dr. Nehi	98
Dr. Pepper	98
Fruit punch	
Shasta	110
Fruit mix	
Wyler's	88
Ginger Ale	
Canada Dry	85
Fanta	85
Nehi	91

1

Beverages

Crush	120
Fanta	114
Hi-C	101
Nedick's	121
Nehi	124
Patio	128
Schweppes	118
Shasta	114
Sunkist	125

Pineapple

Canada Dry	110

Purple Passion

Canada Dry	120

Quinine Water

Canada Dry	95
Fanta	84
Schweppes	88

Rondo

Schweppes	100

Root Beer

A&W	114
Berks County	116
Canada Dry Barrelhead	110
Canada Dry Rooti	110
Dad's	105
Fanta	103
Hires	100
On Tap	105
Patio	110
Royal Crown	113

Schweppes 105

Shasta 100

7-Up 97

Sprite 95

Squirt 91

Strawberry

Canada Dry 120

Crush 121

Fanta 121

Nehi 116

Shasta 94

Yoo-Hoo 124

Sun-Drop 118

Teem 93

Tahitian Treat

Canada Dry 130

Tiki 100

Tonic

Canada Dry 90

Schweppes 88

Shasta 66

Upper 10 101

Vanilla

Yoo-Hoo 125

Vanilla Cream

Canada Dry 130

Wild Cherry

Canada Dry 130

Wink 120

COFFEE AND TEA, 6 oz

Coffee	
regular	2
instant	4
flavored	
General Foods	
Cafe Francais	60
Cafe Vienna	60
Orange Cappuccino	60
Suisse Mocha	60
Postum	10
Tea, bags or loose	1
Tea, bottled or canned	
Lipton	84
sugar free	1
No-Cal	0
Tea, instant	
Lipton lemon-flavored	3
100% Tea	0
Nestea	1
Tender Leaf	1
Tea, mix, iced, lemon-flavored	
Our Own (A&P)	62
Lipton	40
Nestea	15
with sugar	70

Salada	57
Wyler's	56

FRUIT AND VEGETABLE JUICES, 6 oz

Fresh

Grapefruit	70
Lemon or Lime	45
Lemon or Lime, 1 Tbsp	3
Orange	
California	85
Florida	80
Valencia	85
Peach Nectar	90
Tangerine	80

Bottled and Canned

Apple	
Ann Page	90
Heinz	75

Musselman's	80
Mott's	80
Pillsbury	60
Seneca	80
Welch's	90

Apple-Cranberry

Lincoln	104

Apricot nectar

Del Monte	100
Heart's Delight	194
Heinz	104
Libby's	110
Seneca	75

Cranberry-Apple

Cranapple	120

Fig

Real Fig	135

Fig and Prune

Fig 'n' Prune	135

Grape

Heinz	120
Seneca	110
Welch's	120

Grapefruit

Del Monte	70
Heinz	70
Libby's	75
Ocean Spray	70
Seneca	55
Stokely-Van Camp	60

Welch's	75
Grapefruit-Orange	
Seneca	77
Grenadine syrup, nonalcoholic, 1 oz.	
Garnier	100
Giroux	104
Lemon, 1 Tbsp	
ReaLemon	4
Rose's	5
Lime, 1 Tbsp	
ReaLime	6
Orange	
Del Monte	80
Heinz	75
Libby's	90
Welch's	90
Orange-Grapefruit	
Del Monte	80
Libby's	80
Stokely-Van Camp	70
Peach Nectar	
Del Monte	100
Libby's	90
Heart's Delight	89
Pear Nectar	
Del Monte	110
Libby's	100
Heart's Delight	95
Pineapple	
Del Monte	100

1

Dole	93
Heinz	95
Seneca	68
Stokely-Van Camp	110
Pineapple-Grapefruit	
Del Monte	90
Pineapple-Orange	
Ann Page	87
Del Monte	90
Hi-C	94
Lincoln	97
Prune	
Ann Page	140
Del Monte	120
Heinz	130
Mott's	140
RealPrune	130
Seneca	130
Sunsweet	124
Welch's	150
Tomato	
Campbell's	35
Del Monte	35
Heinz	38
Hunt's	43
Libby's	39
Sacramento	32
Seneca	27
Stokely-Van Camp	33
Townhouse	35

Welch's	38
Vegetable	
Campbell V-8	35
Vegemato	32

Frozen Juice

Grape	
Minute Maid	99
Snow Crop	99
Grapefruit	
Bird's Eye	68
Minute Maid	75
Snow Crop	75
Lemon	
Minute Maid	40
Orange	
Bright and Early	90
Minute Maid	90
Snow Crop	120
Stokely-Van Camp	90
Orange-Grapefruit	
Bird's Eye	72
Minute Maid	76
Pineapple	
Dole	101
Minute Maid	92

Pineapple-orange
  Minute Maid   94
  Dole   77
Tangerine
  Minute Maid   86
  Snow Crop   85

Dairy-Packed Juice, 8 oz

Grapefruit
  Tropicana   75
Orange
  Borden   96
  Kraft   90
  Sealtest   96
  Tropicana   83
Orange-Grapefruit
  Kraft   90
Orange-Pineapple
  Ann Page   87
  Hi-C   94
  Kraft   96

1

FRUIT-FLAVORED DRINKS, ALL TYPES, 6 oz

Apple
Ann Page	90
Hi-C	90

Apple-Grape
Mott's	90
Welch's	92

Apricot-Apple
BC	92

Cherry
Ann Page	90
Hi-C	75

Citrus Cooler
Ann Page	90
Hi-C	90

Cranberry
Ann Page	120
Ocean Spray	105
Seneca	120
Welch's	105

Cranberry-Apple
Ann Page	135
Lincoln	103
Mott's	95
Ocean Spray	135

Cranberry-Apricot
  Ocean Spray 105
Cranberry-Grape
  Ocean Spray 105
  Welch's 120
Cranberry-Orange
  Knox 59
Cranberry-Prune
  Ocean Spray 120
Grape
  Ann Page 90
  Hi-C 90
  Welch's 90
Grape-Apple
  BC 107
Grapefruit
  Ann Page 80
  Sealtest 90
  Tropicana 70
Lemon
  Sealtest 90
Lemonade
  Bird's Eye 74
  Borden 78
  Country Time 67
  Hi-C 75
  Minute Maid 75
  ReaLemon 76
  Sealtest 80
  Snow Crop 75

Stokely-Van Camp	80
Wyler's	67

Lemon-Limeade

Minute Maid	75
Snow Crop	75

Limeade

Bird's Eye	75
Minute Maid	75
Snow Crop	75

Orange

A&P	80
Ann Page	90
Bird's Eye	105
Borden	85
Hi-C	125
Minute Maid	125
Start	120
Stokely-Van Camp	114
Tang	120
Tropicana	93
Welch's	135

Orange-Pineapple

Ann Page	120
BC	120
Start	120

Peach

Hi-C	120

Pineapple-Grapefruit

Dole	120

Punch
Ann Page — 120
Hawaiian Punch — 120
Hi-C — 130
Mott's — 120
Stokely-Van Camp — 114
Tropicana — 93
Welch's — 130
Wyler's — 85

Raspberry
Wyler's — 85

Strawberry
Hi-C — 120
Wyler's — 85

Tangerine
Hi-C — 120

Wild Berry
Ann Page — 120
Hi-C — 115

CHAPTER 2

Dairy

BUTTER AND MARGARINE

Butter
  ½ cup (¼ lb)   815
  1 Tbsp   100
Butter, whipped
  ½ cup   540
  1 Tbsp   65
Margarine, 1 Tbsp
  Imitation
    Mazola   50
    Parkay   50
    Weight Watchers   50

Regular and Soft, all brands	100
Diet, all brands	50
Spread	
Blue Bonnet	80
Fleishmann	80
Parkay	70
Whipped, all brands	70

CHEESE, 1 oz unless noted

American	
Borden	104
Kraft	90
Blue	
Borden	105
Casino	100
Kraft	99
Brie	
Dorman	100
Kraft	100
Camembert	
Borden	85
Kraft	85
Caraway	
Kraft	111
Cheddar	
Borden	113
Kraft	113

2

Colby
Borden 111
Kraft 111

Cottage, 1 cup
creamed
Borden 240
Breakstone 230
Breakstone low-fat 180
Foremost 212
Friendship 360
Kraft 214
Lucerne 240
Meadow Gold 134
Sealtest 114
partly creamed
Meadow Gold 204
Sealtest 176
uncreamed, potstyle
Borden 196
Breakstone 170
Kraft 206
Sealtest 180
low fat
Borden 180
Breakstone 180
Friendship 200
Lucerne 200
Viva 200
Weight Watchers 180

Cream cheese
- *Borden*   96
- *Kraft Philadelphia Brand*   98

Edam
- *Dorman*   105
- *House of Gold*   105

Farmer's
- *Breakstone*   30
- *Dutch Garden*   100
- *Friendship*   38
- *Wispride*   100

Fondue
- *Swiss Knight*   60

Fontina
- *Kraft*   114

Frankenmuth
- *Kraft*   113

Gjetost
- *Kraft*   135

Gorgonzola
- *Kraft*   112

Gouda
- *Borden*   86
- *Kraft*   108

Gruyère
- *Borden*   101
- *Kraft*   108
- *Swiss Knight*   101

Leyden
- *Kraft*   80

Liederkranz
   Borden   86

Limburger
   Borden   97
   Dorman   100
   Kraft   98
   Mountain Valley   100

Monterey Jack
   Borden   103
   Casino   100
   Kraft   103

Mozzarella
   Borden   79
   Kraft   79
   Dorman   85

Muenster
   Borden   85
   Dorman   90
   Kraft   100

Neufchâtel
   Borden   73
   Kraft   69

Nuworld
   Kraft   104

Parmesan, grated, 1 Tbsp
   Buitoni   23
   Kraft   27
   La Rosa   33
   Lucerne   25

Parmesan & Romano, grated, 1 Tbsp
Borden   30
Kraft   30

Pimiento
Borden   104
Kraft   104

Port Salut
Dorman   100
Kraft   100

Premost
Kraft   134

Provolone
Borden   93
Kraft   99

Ricotta
Borden   42
Kraft   99

Romano, grated, 1 Tbsp
Buitoni   21
Kraft   26

Roquefort
Borden   107
Kraft   105

Sap Sago
Kraft   76

Sardo Romano
Kraft   110

Scamorze
Kraft   100

Swiss
  Borden   104
  Dorman   90
  Kraft   104
Sage
  Kraft   113
Tilsit
  Dorman   95

Cheese Food

American
  Borden   92
  Kraft   77
Blue
  Borden   82
  Borden Vera Blue   91
  Wispride   100
Cheddar
  Wispride   100
Jalapeno pepper
  Kraft   93
Munst-ett
  Kraft   101
Pimiento
  Borden   91
  Pauley Swiss   90
  Velveeta   90
Pizza
  Kraft   80

Sharp
Kraft 93
Swiss
Borden 91
Kraft 91

Cheese Spread

American
Borden 85
Kraft 77
Kraft Old English 97
American with Bacon
Borden 80
Kraft 92
Blue
Borden 82
Roka 80
Wispride 92
Cheddar
Snack Mate 85
Wispride 97
Garlic
Borden 82
Kraft 86
Limburger
Borden 82

Mohawk Valley	70
Moose	70
Pimiento	
Cheez Whiz	76
Kraft	77
Snack Mate	90
Smoked	
Borden	80
Velveeta	80

CREAM, 1 Tbsp

half and half	
Borden	19
Meadow Gold	27
Sealtest	20
light	
Borden	25
Foremost	30
Sealtest	35
medium	
Borden	41
Sealtest	42
heavy (whipping)	
Borden	52

Foremost	52
Lucerne	10
Sealtest	52

Sour Cream, 1 Tbsp

Borden	29
Borden half and half	29
Borden imitation	25
Foremost	30
Sealtest	29

Non-Dairy Creamers, 1 Tsp

coffee creamers
Carnation Coffee-Mate	11
Meadow Gold	9
Pet Cremora	11

whipped toppings
Reddi-Whip	7
Sta-Whip	8

EGGS

Chicken
  raw, boiled, or poached
    medium   72
    large   82
    extra large   94
  raw, white only
    medium   15
    large   18
    extra large   20
    1 cup   125
  raw, yolk only
    medium   53
    large   60
    extra large   68
  fried
    medium   85
    large   97
    extra large   113
  scrambled or omelet
    medium   99
    large   110
    extra large   127
Duck, raw   130
Goose, raw   266
Turkey, raw   135

Egg Mixes, Commercial

Imitation
Morningstar Farms Scramblers, ½ cup   130
Tillie Lewis Eggstra, 1 pkt   101
Fleishmann Egg Beaters, ½ cup   81
Omelets, 1 pkt
Plain
  Durkee   604
  Durkee dry mix   112
with bacon
  Durkee   620
  Durkee dry mix   125
with cheese
  Durkee   617
  Durkee dry mix   127
  McCormick   130
  Schilling   128
Western
  Durkee   604
  Durkee dry mix   112
  McCormick   115
  Schilling   115
Scrambled
  Durkee   124
with bacon
  Durkee   180
with sausage and potatoes
  Swanson   452

MILK, 8 oz

Buttermilk
  Borden
    .1% fat — 88
    .5% fat — 90
    1% fat — 107
    1.5% fat — 110
    2% fat — 122
    3% fat — 158
  Friendship 1.4% fat — 120
  Golden Nugget .8% — 92
  Light 'n Lively .8% fat — 95
  Lucerne 1.5% fat — 120
  Sealtest 2% fat — 114
Skim
  Borden .1% fat — 81
  Lucerne
    0% fat — 90
    1% fat — 110
    2% fat — 130
  Meadow Gold
    .5% fat — 87
    2% fat — 130
  Sealtest .1% fat — 79
Skim Fortified
  Borden — 81
  Borden Lite Line — 117
  Borden Hi Protein — 132

Gail Borden	81
Light 'n Lively	114
Sealtest	137
Whole	
Borden	160
Foremost	154
Lucerne	160
Meadow Gold	166
Sealtest	150
Whole Fortified	
Gail Borden	159
Sealtest Multivitamin	151

Milk Beverages, 8 oz unless noted

Cherry-vanilla	
Borden	291
Chocolate	
Borden	210
Meadow Gold	190
Sealtest	175
Chocolate fudge	
Borden	284
Chocolate mixes	
Carnation Instant, 1 pkt	130
Carnation Slender, 1 pkt	110
Nestle's Quik	215

2

Ovaltine, 1 oz	105
Pillsbury, 1 pkt	295
Safeway, 2 tsp	215
Sealtest	195

Chocolate malt mix

Carnation Instant, 1 pkt	130
Carnation Slender, 1 pkt	110

Eggnog, dairy packed

Borden

4.7% fat	260
6% fat	302
8% fat	375
Carnation, 1 pkt	130
Meadow Gold	327
Sealtest	324

Malt

Borden	80
Carnation	90
Ovaltine	100

Mocha

Borden	291

Strawberry

Borden	287
Carnation, 1 pkt	130
Pillsbury, 1 pkt	290

Vanilla

Borden	291
Carnation, 1 pkt	130

YOGURT, 8 oz

Plain
Borden Lite-Line	140
Borden Swiss Style	167
Breakstone	144
Dannon	150
Light 'n Lively	140
Lucerne	160
Pet	157
Viva	180

Flavored, all flavors
Borden	270
Breyer's	270
Dannon	210
Light 'n Lively	240
Meadow Gold	270
Viva	250

Frozen
Danny
In-A-Cup, 8 oz.	180
On-A-Stick, uncoated	65

CHAPTER 3

Breads, Crackers, Flour

BREAD, 1 slice, approximately 1 oz unless noted

Tasty Bake 70

Date Nut
Thomas 100

French
Pepperidge Farm 79
Wonder 75

Garlic
Stouffer 80

Gluten
Thomas 32

Hollywood 70

Honey Bran
Pepperidge Farm 58

Honey Wheatberry
Arnold 90
Pepperidge Farm 60

Italian
Pepperidge Farm 81

Naturel
Arnold 65

Nut
Brownberry 85

Oatmeal
Brownberry 82
Pepperidge Farm 66

Profile 52

Protein
Thomas 45

Pumpernickel
Arnold 75

Pepperidge Farm	79
Raisin	
Plain	
Arnold	75
Thomas	66
with cinnamon	
Brownberry	85
Pepperidge Farm	75
Thomas	65
with nuts	
Brownberry	95
Rice Cakes	
Spiral	36
Rye	
Arnold	50
Jewish	75
soft	75
Brownberry	65
Pepperidge Farm	82
Tasty Bake	91
Wonder	75
Sourdough	
Di Carlo	71
Wheat	
Arnold	
Granary	71
Branola	90
Brick Oven	60
Melba Thin	40
Brownberry	85

3

Buckwheat 75
Colonial 72
Home Pride 75
Pepperidge Farm 70
Pepperidge Farm Very Thin 40
Thomas 50
Wonder 75
Wheat Germ
Pepperidge Farm 69
White
Arnold
  Brick Oven, .8 oz slice 65
  Brick Oven, 1.1 oz slice 85
  Country 95
  Hearthstone Country 70
  Melba Thin 40
Brownberry Sandwich 75
Brownberry Thin 70
Butternut 75
Colonial 75
Daffodil Farm 58
Fresh Horizons 50
Hart 75
Heartstone 85
Home Pride 75
Homestyle 75
Manor 75
Pepperidge Farm 75
Pepperidge Farm Sandwich 72
Sweetheart 75

Tasty Bake	72
Thomas	64
Weight Watchers	35
Wonder	75
Whole Wheat	
Pepperidge Farm	61
Thomas	65

Bread, Canned, ½ inch slice

Banana Nut	
Dromedary	71
Brown	
B&M	52
Chocolate Nut	
Cross & Blackwell	65
Dromedary	87
Date Nut	
Dromedary	75
Fruit and Nut	
Cross & Blackwell	77
Orange Nut	
Cross & Blackwell	76
Dromedary	78
Spice Nut	
Cross & Blackwell	65

3

Bread Mixes

White, ¼ loaf	
Pillsbury	460
Cornbread, 1 pkg	
Pillsbury	320
Aunt Jemima	330

BISCUITS, MUFFINS AND ROLLS

Biscuits, Baking Powder, 1 biscuit

1869 Brand	105
prebaked	100
Pillsbury	70
Tenderflake	60

Biscuits, refrigerated, 1 biscuit

Plain	
Ballard	50
Borden	59
Hungry Jack	95
Flaky	90

Pillsbury	55
Flaky Baking Powder	67
Tenderflake	
Baking Powder	60
Buttermilk	
Hungry Jack	
Extra Rich	65
Flaky	80
Fluffy	100
Pillsbury	50
Big Country	95
Extra Light	55
Tenderflake	55
Corn Bread	
Pillsbury	95

Muffins, frozen, 1 muffin

Blueberry	
Thomas	110
Howard Johnson	121
Morton	120
Rounds	110
Pepperidge Farm	130
Corn	
Howard Johnson	118
Morton	
regular	130

Rounds	125
Pepperidge Farm	140
Thomas	120
English	
Thomas	130
Orange	
Howard Johnson	115
Raisin Bran	
Pepperidge Farm	130

Muffins, Mix, 1 muffin

Apple Cinnamon	
Betty Crocker	160
Banana Nut	
Betty Crocker	185
Blueberry	
Betty Crocker	120
Corn	
Betty Crocker	160
Orange	
Betty Crocker	155
Pineapple	
Betty Crocker	125

Muffins, packaged

Bran
  Thomas — 118
Cinnamon Raisin
  Pepperidge Farm — 140
Corn
  Thomas — 180
  Toast-r-Cakes — 120
English
  Di Carlo — 145
  Hostess — 145
  Thomas — 140
  Wonder — 144
Honey Butter
  Arnold Orowheat — 150
Onion
  Thomas — 130
Raisin
  Wonder — 155
Sourdough
  Wonder — 130
Wheat
  Home Pride — 140

3

Muffins, refrigerated, 1 muffin

Apple Cinnamon
Pillsbury   155
Corn
Pillsbury   130

Rolls, 1 roll

Hard Rolls
Pepperidge Farm   120
   French, 3 oz   264
   French, 5 oz   395
   Hearth   64
   Sesame Crisp   76
Wonder   82
Sandwich and Hamburger Rolls
Arnold
   Dutch Egg Buns   130
   Francisco   180
   Soft   110
   Hamburger   110
   Hot Dog   110
Colonial   160
Pepperidge Farm   120
Wonder   160
Soft Rolls
Arnold

Deli-Twist	110
Finger, 24's and 12's	55
Francisco	100
Refrigerator	95
Ballard	95
Borden	
Gem Flake	70
Onion	95
Colonial	80
Home Pride	90
Pepperidge Farm	
Butter Crescent	130
Dinner	65
Finger	60
Golden Twist	120
Old Fashioned	37
Parkerhouse	60
Party	35
Pillsbury	
Butterflake	110
Crescent	95
Hot Roll Mix	95
Wonder	
Buttermilk	85
Pan	105
Sweet Rolls, refrigerated	
Caramel	
Pillsbury	160
Cinnamon	
Ballard	100

Hungry Jack	145
Pillsbury	114
Orange	
Pillsbury	130
Scones	
Hostess	188

CRACKERS, 1 piece

Bacon Flavored
Keebler	15
Nabisco Bacon Thins	11

Barbecue
Chit Chat	14
Sunshine	17

Butter
Hi-Ho	17
Keebler	
Butter Thins	17
Club	15
Townhouse	19
Nabisco	15
Ritz	17
Tam-Tams	13

Butter-cheese
Ritz	18

Caraway
Caraway Crazy	15

Cheese
Cheese-Nips	5
Cheese Tid-Bits	4
Cheez-It	6
Che-Zo	5
Keebler	11
Pepperidge Farm	12

Cheese-peanut Butter
Keebler	14

Chicken
Chicken In a Biskit	10

Club
Keebler	15

Flings Curls
Nabisco	10

Gold Fish
Pepperidge Farm, 1 oz	140

Ham
Nabisco	12

Hi-Ho
Sunshine	18

Kavli Flatbread 35

Matzos
Goodman's Square	110
Goodman's Tea	75
Horowitz-Margareten	130
Manischewitz	
Egg	132

Egg 'N Onion	113
Regular	110
Tam Tams	14
Tasteas	115
Thin Tea	110
Whole Wheat	122

Onion
Keebler	15
Manischewitz	13
Nabisco	13
French Onion	12
Pepperidge Farm	12

Potato
Chippers	14
Potato Piffles	17

Ritz
Nabisco	17

Rye
Keebler Rye Toast	18
Peek Frean	30
Ry Krisp	24

Saltines
Jacob's	
Biscuits for Cheese	35
English Cream	110
Keebler	
Salt-Free	15
Saltines	14
Sea Toast	60
Whole Wheat Sea Toast	58

Nabisco
Premium 12
Royal Lunch 54
Uneeda 22
Sunshine 11

Sesame
Keebler 16
Meal Mates 22
Sesame Sillys 15
Sunshine 24

Shapies 10

Sip'N Chips 10

Sociables
Nabisco 10

Toasts
Dutch Rusk 60
Holland Rusk 39
Keebler 15
Old London 11
Pepperidge Farm 11
Sunshine All-Rye 21

Soda and water crackers
Huntley & Palmer 35
Jacob's Golden Puffs 34
Keebler Milk Lunch 27
Waldorf 18
Zesta 14

Tomato-onion
Sunshine 15

Town House
Keebler   15
Triangle Thins
Nabisco   8
Twig:
Nabisco   14
Waffle crackers   22
Waverly wafers
Nabisco   18
Wheat
Nabisco
Wheat Toast   15
Wheat Thins   9
Zwieback
Nabisco   31

OTHER BREAD PRODUCTS

Breadcrumbs, 1 cup   450

Contadina   450
4C plain   410
4C seasoned   400

Breadsticks, 1 piece

onion
  Stella D'Oro   35
plain
  Stella D'Oro   40
sesame
  Stella D'Oro   38
dietetic
  Stella D'Oro   43

Croutons, ½ cup unless noted

bacon
  Bel Air   80
  Brownberry   90
cheese and garlic
  Bel Air   100
garlic
  Bel Air   80
Italian cheese
  Bel Air   100
plain
  Bel Air   60
seasoned
  Bel Air   90
  Brownberry   90

3

Stuffing, mixes, 1 pkg

Pepperidge Farm	110
Stove Top	170
Uncle Ben's	120

FLOURS, 1 cup

Buckwheat	
dark	325
light	340
Cake	370
Carob	250
Corn	485
Corn Starch, 1 Tbsp	35
Lima Bean	430
Peanut	225
Rye	
light	315
medium	310
dark	420
Soybean, defatted	325
full fat	300
low fat	310
Tortilla	
corn	410

wheat	450
Wheat, all purpose	485
bread	500
cake	430
gluten	530
self-rising	440
whole wheat	400
White	400
Unbleached	400

Meal, 1 cup

Almond	696
Corn	433
Cracker	450
Graham cracker	465
Matzo	444

CHAPTER 4

Cereal, Pancakes, Waffles and French Toast

CEREAL, ready to eat, 1 cup

bran

All-Bran, *Kellogg's*	190
40% Bran Flakes, *Kellogg's*	140
100% Bran Flakes, *Nabisco*	150
40% Bran Flakes, *Post*	125
Bran Chex, *Ralston Purina*	165
Bran & Prune Flakes, *Post*	120
Bran & Raisin Flakes, *General Mills*	125
Raisin Bran, *Kellogg's*	200
Raisin Bran, *Ralston Purina*	200
Raisin Bran, *Safeway*	200

Raisin Bran with Sugar Coating, *Post*   178
Bran-Buds with wheat germ, *Kellogg's*   200

corn

Country Corn Flakes, *General Mills*   80
Kix, *General Mills*   75
Corn Flakes, *Kellogg's*   110
Toasties Corn Flakes, *Post*   110
Corn Chex, *Ralston Purina*   110
Corn Flakes, *Ralston Purina*   110
Corn Flakes, *Safeway*   110
Corn Flakes & Blueberries, *Post*   110
Corn Flakes & Strawberries, *Post*   110
Sugar Frosted Flakes, *Kellogg's*   144
Sugar Pops, *Kellogg's*   105
Honeycomb Corn, *Post*   85
Sugar Sparkled Flakes, *Post*   149
Cocoa Puffs, *General Mills*   110
Trix, *General Mills*   111

corn and oats

Sugar Sparkled Twinkies, *General Mills*   112
Cap'n Crunch, *Quaker*   163
Crisp, *Quaker*   105

oats

Cheerios, *General Mills*   110
OK's, *Kellogg's*   83
Alpha-Bits, *Post*   110
Crispy Critters, *Post*   110
Fortified Oat Flakes, *Post*   165
Life, *Quaker*   160
Lucky Charms, *General Mills*   110

Frosty O's, *General Mills*	110
Sugar Jets, *General Mills*	111
Stars, *Kellogg's*	112
Fruit Loops, *Kellogg's*	112

rice

Rice Krispies, *Kellogg's*	105
Puffed Rice, *Quaker*	45
Crispy Rice, *Ralston Purina*	110
Rice Chex, *Ralston*	110
Crispy Rice, *Safeway*	110
Puffa Puffa Rice, *Kellogg's*	120
Rice Honeys, *Nabisco*	150
Rice Krinkles, *Post*	127
Cocoa Crispies, *Kellogg's*	113

wheat

Buc Wheats, *General Mills*	146
Total, *General Mills*	110
Wheat Stax, *General Mills*	81
Wheaties, *General Mills*	108
Crumbles, *Kellogg's*	140
Pep, *Kellogg's*	106
Shredded Wheat, *Kellogg's* 1 biscuit	63
Shredded Wheat, *Nabisco* 1 biscuit	92
Grape Nuts Flakes, *Post*	150
Puffed Wheat, *Quaker*	38
Shredded Wheat, *Quaker* 1 biscuit	68
Wheat Chex, *Ralston Purina*	165
Sugar Crisp, *Kellogg's*	147
Sugar Smacks, *Kellogg's*	110
Wheat Honeys, *Nabisco*	153

4

mixed grains

Concentrate, *Kellogg's*	310
Product 19, *Kellogg's*	106
Special K, *Kellogg's*	70
Apple Jacks, *Kellogg's*	112
Team Flakes, *Nabisco*	83
Grape Nuts, *Post*	400
Quake, *Quaker*	118

Cereal, cooked, 1 cup

barley
Quaker	172

corn meal mush
Quaker	128

farina

Cream of Wheat
Instant	133
Mix'N Eat	140
Quick	133
Regular	133
H-O	168
Pillsbury	120
Quaker	100

grits

Quaker
Instant	79

Instant with cheese flavor, 1 pkt	105
Instant with imitation bacon, 1 pkt	100
Instant with imitation ham, 1 pkt	100
3-Minute Brand, ¼ cup	150
oats	
H-O	150
Quaker	160
oatmeal	
Quaker	143
rice	
Cream of Rice	145
rye	
Con Agra	360
whole wheat	
Quaker Pettilohns	145

PANCAKES, FRENCH TOAST, WAFFLES AND OTHER BREAKFASTS, 1 piece unless noted

Breakfast Bars, frozen

Carnation	210
General Mills	190

Crepes, mix, 6″ crepe
Aunt Jemima	55

French Toast, frozen
Aunt Jemima	85
with cinnamon	100
Downyflake	135
Swanson, with sausage, 1 pkg	335

French Toast, mix
McCormick	119

Fritters, frozen
Mrs. Paul's	120

Pancakes, frozen
Downyflake	75
Swanson, with sausage, 1 pkg	500

Pancakes, frozen batter
Aunt Jemima	70

Pancakes, mix, 4″ pancake
Aunt Jemima	
Easy Pour	60
buckwheat	80
buttermilk	70
Betty Crocker	70
Hungry Jack	75
blueberry	112
buttermilk	80
Extra Lights	60

Pancake-Waffle, mix
Aunt Jemima	70
buttermilk	100
whole wheat	80

Log Cabin	60
buttermilk	75
Waffle, mix	
Aunt Jemima	100
Downyflake	60
Jumbo	89

CHAPTER 5

Beans, Pasta and Rice

BARLEY, 1 cup

pearled, light	698
pearled, Pot or Scotch	696

BEANS DRIED,
1 cup unless noted

Broadbeans, raw, immature seeds, 8 oz	238
Broadbeans, raw, mature seeds, 8 oz	768

5

Black, dry, uncooked, 8 oz	768
Chick peas	
8 oz	817
1 cup	720
Great Northern	212
Lima, immature seeds	190
Lima, mature seeds, dried	262
Mung, dried	714
Pea or Navy, dried	224
Pinto (red Mexican), uncooked	663
Red Kidney	220
White, dried	224

Baked Beans, ½ cup

B & M	180
Campbell	148
barbecue	171
with franks	181
with pork	147
Heinz	140
Campside	180
with franks	184
with pork	150
Howard Johnson's	163
Morton House	160

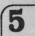
PASTA, 1 cup unless noted

Dry

egg noodles
Goodman's	175
La Rosa	190
La Rosa spinach	200
Pennsylvania Dutch	200
Prince	190
Ronzoni	200

macaroni
Goodman's	170
La Rosa	180
Prince	170
Ronzoni	175

spaghetti
Buitoni	175
Goodman's	160
La Rosa	165
Prince	160
Ronzoni	165

5

Macaroni, canned, bagged, frozen and mixes

with beef
Banquet	260
Chef Boy-Ar-Dee	235
Franco-American	220
Green Giant Boil-in-Bag, 1 pkg	240
Morton	260
Stouffer's, 1 pkg	380

with beef and cheese
Banquet	300
Green Giant Boil-in-Bag, 1 pkg	330
Hormel, 7½ oz can	340
Howard Johnson's	330
Morton	215
Mac-A-Roni & Cheddar	290
Pennsylvania Dutch	310
Stouffer's, 1 pkg	520
Swanson	200

with cheese sauce
Franco-American	225
Heinz	230
MacaroniO's	180
Noodle-Roni	290
Scallop-A-Roni	275

with chili sauce
Fiesta Mac-A-Roni	270

creole style
Heinz, 8¾-oz can	169

Noodles, canned, frozen and mixes

Almondine
Betty Crocker, 1 pkg | 960
with beef
Heinz, 8½ oz can | 170
with beef in gravy
College Inn | 238
with beef in tomato sauce
College Inn | 238
with beef
Hormel, 7½-oz can | 240
with beef sauce
Pennsylvania Dutch | 260
Betty Crocker | 170
with butter sauce
Pennsylvania Dutch | 300
with cheese
Noodle-Roni | 650
with cheese sauce
Pennsylvania Dutch | 300
with cheese sauce and sour cream
Noodle-Roni Romanoff | 362
with chicken
Dinty Moore, 7½-oz can | 215
with chicken sauce
Noodle-Roni | 250
Pennsylvania Dutch | 300
Twist-A-Roni | 250

Romanoff
Betty Crocker, 1 pkg	800
Stouffer's, 1 pkg	500

Stroganoff
Betty Crocker, 1 pkg	900
Pennsylvania Dutch	630

with tuna
Stouffer's, 1 pkg	400

Noodles, Italian style, canned, frozen and mixes

Cannelloni, 8 oz
Weight Watchers	275

Eggplant Parmigiana, 8 oz
Buitoni	421
Weight Watchers	172

Lasagna, 8 oz unless noted
Buitoni	250
with meat sauce	340
Chef Boy-Ar-Dee	
canned	241
mix	265
Golden Grain, 1 pkg	720
Green Giant	
Boil-in-Bag, 1 pkg	310
Oven Bake, 1 pkg	300
Hormel	
7½-oz can	270
10-oz can	370

Lean Cuisine, 11 oz	260
Lean Line, 10 oz	270
Roman	274
Stouffer's, 1 pkg	385
Swanson, 1 pkg	540
Weight Watchers	215

Manicotti, 8 oz
Buitoni	395
with sauce	350
Lean Line	270

Ravioli, 8 oz
Buitoni
cheese	575
meat	680

Chef Boy-Ar-Dee
cheese	263
meat	210

Franco-American, 7½-oz can	220

La Rosa
cheese	205
meat	218

Roman
cheese	496
meat	552

Ravioli Parmigiana, 8 oz
Buitoni
cheese	301
meat	381

5

Rotini
Franco-American, 7½-oz can 200
    with meatballs 230

Shells
Buitoni, 8 oz 235
Lean Line, 11 oz 270

Spaghetti, all with tomato sauce, 1 cup unless noted
Banquet with meatballs 212
Betty Crocker, 1 pkg 170
Buitoni
    with meatballs 250
    with mushrooms 170
Chef Boy-Ar-Dee
    with cheese sauce 180
    with meat 260
    with meat sauce 250
    with meatballs 250
    with mushrooms 225
Franco-American
    with cheese sauce 200
    with meat 290
    with meatballs 260
Spaghetti-Os
    with cheese 200
    with meatballs 228
Golden Grain 275
Green Giant, Boil-in-Bag
    with meatballs 280

Heinz
   with cheese sauce   175
   with franks   310
   with meat sauce   173
Hormel
   with meat   280
   with meat sauce   205
Kraft   260
La Rosa with meatballs   230
Lean Cuisine   280
Libby's with meatballs   95
Morton, frozen, 1 pkg   220
Stouffer's, 1 pkg   445
Swanson, 1 pkg   290

Ziti

Buitoni, 8 oz   270
Lean Line, 10 oz   270
Weight Watchers, 1 pkg   350

RICE, 1 cup unless noted

Plain

Ann Page, whole pkg   1000
Bird's Eye   260
Carolina   200

Green Giant	230
Minute	300
Rice-A-Roni, whole pkg	780
River	200
Uncle Ben's	200
Uncle Ben's, brown	250

Flavored

beef
    Uncle Ben's   210

beef and cracked rice
    Betty Crocker   416

beef and vermicelli
    Minute   300
    Rice-A-Roni   315

beef and cheese sauce
    Betty Crocker   350

chicken
    Uncle Ben's   210

chicken with crumb topping
    Betty Crocker   365

chicken and vermicelli
    Minute   300
    Rice-A-Roni   321

curry
    Uncle Ben's   205

fried Chinese and vermicelli
    Rice-A-Roni   375

ham and vermicelli
    Rice-A-Roni   300

pilaf
  Uncle Ben's   290
Frozen
  Green Giant   160
    Medley   220
    Pilaf   240
    Verdi   140
Spanish, canned
  Heinz   190
  La Rosa   155
  Libby's   57
  Stokely-Van Camp   180

Bulgur (parboiled wheat), 1 cup

Club Wheat, dry   630
Hard Red Winter Wheat, dry   605
  canned, unseasoned   225
  seasoned   246
White Wheat, dry   555

CHAPTER 6

Soup

CANNED OR FROZEN,
1 cup unless noted

Alphabet
Golden Grain   55
Alphabet vegetable
Lipton   68
Asparagus, cream of
Campbell's   165
Bean
  plain
  Manischewitz   112
  Wyler's   95

with bacon
Ann Page	140
Campbell's	174
Town House	155

with hot dogs
Campbell's	168

with smoked pork
Heinz	160

Bean, black
Campbell's	95
Crosse & Blackwell	118

Bean, lima
Manischewitz	93

Beef

plain
Campbell's	105
Lipton	200

with barley
Manischewitz	83
Wyler's	72

with cabbage
Manischewitz	62

with low sodium
Campbell's, 7¼-oz can	170

mushroom
Lipton	45

with noodles
Campbell's	69
Heinz	74
Manischewitz	65

Lipton	67
Souptime, 1 envelope	30
Town House	75
Wyler's	50
with vegetables	
Manischewitz	61
Borscht	
Manischewitz	72
Rokeach	75
Bouillon, 1 cube	
beef	
Herb-Ox	6
Knorr-Swiss	15
Maggi	6
Wyler's	7
chicken	
Herb-Ox	6
Knorr-Swiss	17
Maggi	7
Wyler's	8
onion	
Herb-Ox	10
Wyler's	8
vegetable	
Herb-Ox	6
Wyler's	6
Bouillon, instant, 1 tsp	
beef	
Maggi	6
Wyler's	10

chicken
   Maggi   7
   Wyler's   6

Broth
beef
   Campbell's   26
   College Inn   15
   Swanson, 6¾-oz can   25
   Weight Watchers, 1 pkt   10
chicken
   Campbell's   43
   College Inn   32
   Richardson & Robbins   17
   Swanson, 6¼-oz can   25
chicken with noodles
   College Inn   45
chicken with rice
   College Inn   45
   Richardson & Robbins   45

Celery, cream of
   Ann Page   60
   Campbell's   160
   Heinz   180
   Town House   100

Cheddar cheese
   Campbell's   150

Chickarina
   Progresso   100

Chicken
   Lipton   220

Chicken alphabet
  Campbell's — 88
Chicken with barley
  Manischewitz — 83
Chicken, cream of
  Ann Page — 90
  Lipton — 106
  Souptime, 1 pkt — 100
  Town House — 95
Chicken with dumplings
  Campbell's — 100
Chicken gumbo
  Campbell's — 59
Chicken with kasha
  Manischewitz — 41
Chicken with low sodium
  Campbell's, 7½-oz can — 170
Chicken noodle
  A & P — 67
  Ann Page — 70
  Campbell's — 66
  Golden Grain — 74
  Heinz — 35
  Lipton — 54
  Manischewitz — 46
  Souptime, 1 pkt — 30
  Town House — 75
  Wyler's — 44
Chicken with rice
  Ann Page — 50

Campbell's	51
Heinz	58
Lipton	59
Manischewitz	48
Town House	60
Wyler's	49
Chicken with stars	
Ann Page	65
Campbell's	60
Chicken with vegetables	
Ann Page	80
Campbell's	73
Heinz	85
Lipton	70
Manischewitz	55
Town House	85
Wyler's, mix	28
Chili, with beef	
Campbell's	165
Heinz	160
Town House	160
Chowder	
clam, Manhattan	
Campbell's	77
Doxsee	62
Heinz	74
Howard Johnson's	104
Crosse & Blackwell	75
clam, New England	
Campbell's	206

6

Mushroom
Plain
  Campbell's   80
  Golden Grain   95
  Souptime   80
  Wyler's   151
with barley
  Manischewitz   72
bisque
  Crosse & Blackwell   127
cream of
  Ann Page   120
  Campbell's   217
  Heinz   200
  Knorr-Swiss   116
  Lipton   92
  Town House   124
  Wyler's   151

Noodle
  Lipton   50
with chicken broth
  Ann Page, 1 pkt   225
  Lipton   60
with ground beef
  Campbell's   98

Onion
  Ann Page, 1 pkt   125
  Crosse & Blackwell   57
  Golden Grain   33

Knorr-Swiss	45
Lipton	35
Souptime, 1 pkt	20
Wyler's	146
Onion with mushroom	
Lipton	35
Oriental style	
Lipton	210
Oyster stew	
Campbell's	
canned	146
frozen	196
Pea	
green	
Campbell's	148
Golden Grain	73
Knorr-Swiss	71
Lipton	136
Souptime low sodium, 1 pkt	70
with ham	
Campbell's	130
low sodium, 7½-oz can	150
split	
Manischewitz	133
split with ham	
Ann Page	180
Campbell's	180
Heinz	150
Town House	154

Pepper pot
    Campbell's   105
Petite Marmite
    Crosse & Blackwell   41
Potato
  Plain
    Lipton   100
  cream of
    Campbell's   190
  with leek
    Wyler's   155
Schav
    Manischewitz   11
    Rokeach   12
Scotch broth
    Campbell's   90
Senegalese
    Crosse & Blackwell   75
Shrimp, cream of
    Crosse & Blackwell   113
    Campbell's   230
Sirloin burger
    Campbell's   177
Steak and potato
    Campbell's   160
Stockpot
  vegetable
    Lipton   220
  vegetable-beef
    Campbell's   96

6

Tomato

    Ann Page   80
    Campbell's   84
    Heinz   87
    Lipton   93
    Manischewitz   61
    Progresso   110
    Souptime, 1 pkt   70
    Town House   87

Tomato bisque

    Campbell's   126

Tomato

low sodium
    Campbell's 7¼-oz can   130
with rice
    Ann Page   90
    Campbell's   106
    Manischewitz   78
with vegetables
    Golden Grain   86
    Lipton   69

Tuna Creole

    Crosse & Blackwell   70

Turkey

Plain
    Campbell's   138
with noodles
    Ann Page   75

Heinz	83
Lipton	74
Town House	83
low sodium	
Campbell's, 7¼-oz can	60
with vegetables	
Ann Page	60
Campbell's	78
Vegetable	
Plain	
Ann Page	70
Campbell's	83
Old Fashioned	74
Lipton	70
Italian	100
Knorr-Swiss	56
Manischewitz	63
Town House	83
Wyler's	81
with beef	
Ann Page	80
Campbell's	81
low sodium, 7¼-oz can	80
Old Fashioned	79
Heinz	66
Lipton	53
Town House	66
cream of	
Souptime, 1 pkt	80

Soup

Vegetarian
Vichyssoise

CHAPTER 7

Meat, Poultry and Seafood

MEAT, FRESH

Retail cuts of meat are frequently weighed with bone first, *then* they are trimmed, cooked and weighed for their yield. So for instance 1 lb. of pork loin chops are weighed raw with bone, but after they are trimmed and cooked, their yield is 5.9 oz.

Beef, choice-grade, retail cuts

Chuck, arm, roast, or steak; boneless, lean with fat
  raw, 1 lb   1,012
  braised, drained
    10.7 oz (yield from 1 lb)   879
    4 oz   328
    1 cup, chopped   405
    1 cup, ground   318
Chuck, arm, roast, or steak, lean only
  braised, drained
    9.1 oz (yield from 1 lb)   498
    4 oz   219
    1 cup, chopped   270
    1 cup, diced   212
Chuck, rib roast or steak, lean with fat
  raw, 1 lb   1,597
  braised, drained
    10.7 oz (yield from 1 lb)   1,298
    4 oz   484
    1 cup, chopped   598
    1 cup, ground   470
Chuck, stewing; boneless, lean with fat
  raw, 1 lb   1,166
  stewed, drained
    10.7 oz (yield from 1 lb)   994
    4 oz   371
    1 cup, chopped   458
Chuck, stewing; boneless, lean only
  raw, 1 lb   717

stewed, drained

10.7 oz (yield from 1 lb)	651
4 oz	243
1 cup, chopped	300

Club steak, 16% bone, lean with fat

raw, 1 lb	1,443

broiled

9.8 oz (yield from 1 lb raw)	1,262
4 oz without bone	515

Club steak, 16% bone, lean only
broiled

5.7 oz (yield from 1 lb)	393
4 oz without bone	277

Flank steak, boneless, lean only

raw, 1 lb	653

braised, drained

10.7 oz (yield from 1 lb)	596
4 oz	222

Ground, lean with 10% fat

raw, 1 lb	812
broiled, 12 oz (yield from 1 lb)	745

Ground, lean with 21% fat

raw, 1 lb	1,216
broiled, 11.5 oz (yield from 1 lb)	932

Plate, boneless, lean with fat

raw, 1 lb	1,216

simmered, drained

10.7 oz (yield from 1 lb)	1,313
4 oz	490

7

Plate, boneless, lean only
  simmered, drained
    6.5 oz (yield from 1 lb)   368
    4 oz   226

Porterhouse steak, 9% bone, lean with fat
  raw, 1 lb   1,603
  broiled
    10.6 oz (yield from 1 lb)   1,400
    4 oz without bone   527

Porterhouse steak, 9% bone, lean only
  broiled
    6.1 oz (yield from 1 lb)   385
    4 oz without bone   254

Rib roast, boneless, lean with fat
  raw, 1 lb   1,819
  roasted
    11.7 oz (yield from 1 lb)   1,456
    4 oz   499
    1 cup, chopped   616
    1 cup, ground   484

Rib roast, boneless, lean only
  roasted
    7.5 oz (yield from 1 lb)   511
    4 oz   273
    1 cup, chopped   337
    1 cup, ground   265

Round steak, boneless, lean with fat
  raw, 1 lb   894
  braised or broiled
    11.1 oz (yield from 1 lb)   820

4 oz	296

Round steak, boneless, lean only
braised or broiled

9.5 oz (yield from 1 lb)	507
4 oz	296

Rump roast, boneless, lean with fat

raw, 1 lb	1,374

roasted

11.7 oz (yield from 1 lb)	1,149
4 oz	394
1 cup, chopped	486
1 cup, ground	382

Rump roast, boneless, lean only
roasted

8.8 oz (yield from 1 lb)	516
4 oz	236
1 cup, chopped	291
1 cup, ground	229

Sirloin steak, double bone, 18% bone, lean with fat

raw, 1 lb	1,240

broiled

9.6 oz (yield from 1 lb)	1,110
4 oz without bone	463

Sirloin steak, double bone, 18% bone, lean only
broiled

6.3 oz (yield from 1 lb)	372
4 oz without bone	272

Sirloin steak, round-bone, 7% bone, lean with fat

raw, 1 lb	1,316

broiled

10.9 oz (yield from 1 lb)	1,192
4 oz without bone	439

Sirloin steak, round-bone, 7% bone, lean only
broiled

7.2 oz (yield from 1 lb)	420
4 oz without bone	235

T-bone steak, 11% bone, lean with fat

raw, 1 lb	1,596

broiled

10.4 oz (yield from 1 lb)	1,395
4 oz without bone	537

T-bone steak, 11% bone, lean only
broiled

5.8 oz (yield from 1 lb)	368
4 oz without bone	253

Beef, prepared and specialty cuts

Beef, corned

raw, 1 lb	1,596

cooked

10.7 oz (yield from 1 lb)	1,131
4 oz	422

Beef, dried, creamed, home recipe

8 oz	350

Beef, hearts, lean only
raw

8 oz	245

braised	
4 oz	213
1 cup, chopped	273
Beef, kidneys	
raw, 8 oz	294
braised	
4 oz	286
1 cup, chunks	353
Beef, liver	
raw, 1 lb	635
fried, 4 oz	260
Beef pancreas, raw, 4 oz	
fat	358
medium fat	321
lean	160
Beef suet, raw, 1 oz	242
Beef sweetbreads (thymus)	
yearlings, raw, 1 lb	939
yearlings, braised, 4 oz	365
Beef, tongue	
very fat, raw, trimmed, 8 oz	615
fat, raw, trimmed, 8 oz	524
medium-fat, raw, trimmed	
8 oz	470
braised, 4 oz	277
Beef, tripe, 4 oz	
commercial	113
pickled	70

7

Lamb, fresh

Leg, lean with fat
  raw, with bone, 1 lb   845
  roasted, with bone
    9.4 oz (yield from 1 lb)   745
  raw, boneless, 1 lb   1,007
  roasted, boneless
    11.2 oz (yield from 1 lb)   887
    4 oz   317
    1 cup, chopped   391
Leg, lean
  roasted, with bone
    7.8 oz (yield from 1 lb with fat)   411
  roasted, boneless
    9.7 oz (yield from 1 lb with fat)   491
    4 oz   211
    1 cup, chopped   260
Loin chops, with bone, lean with fat
  raw, 1 lb   1,146
  broiled
    10.1 oz (yield from 1 lb)   1,023
    4 oz   407
    1 chop, 3.4 oz   341
    1 chop, 2.5 oz   255
Loin chops, with bone, lean only
  broiled
    6.9 oz (yield from 1 lb)   368
    4 oz   213
    1 chop, 2.3 oz   122

1 chop, 1.7 oz	92
Rib chops with bone, lean with fat	
raw, 1 lb	1,229
broiled	
9.5 oz (yield from 1 lb)	1,091
4 oz	462
1 chop, 3.1 oz	362
1 chop, 2.4 oz	273
Rib chops with bone, lean only	
broiled	
6 oz (yield from 1 lb)	361
4 oz	239
1 chop, 2 oz	120
1 chop, 1.5 oz	91
Shoulder, lean with fat	
raw with bone, 1 lb	1,082
roasted, with bone	
9.5 oz (yield from 1 lb)	913
raw, boneless, 1 lb	1,275
roasted, boneless	
11.2 oz (yield from 1 lb)	1,075
4 oz	383
1 cup, chopped	473
Shoulder, lean only	
roasted, with bone	
7 oz (yield from 1 lb)	410
roasted, boneless	
8.3 oz (yield from 1 lb)	482
4 oz	233
1 cup, chopped	287

7

Lamb's quarters

raw, trimmed, 1 lb	195
boiled, drained	
4 oz	36
1 cup	64

Lamb hearts

raw, 8 oz	368
braised	
4 oz	295
1 cup, chopped	377

Lamb kidneys

raw, 8 oz	238

Lamb liver

raw, 1 lb	617
broiled, 4 oz	296

Lamb tongue

raw, trimmed, 8 oz	452
braised, 4 oz	288

Lamb sweetbreads (thymus), 4 oz

raw	106
braised	200

Ham, retail cuts (see also Pork)

Boiled, 8 oz (about 8 slices)	531
Fresh, lean with fat	
raw, 1 lb with bone and skin	1,188

baked
9.2 oz (yield from 1 lb)	980
raw, 1 lb without bone and skin	1,397

baked
10.9 oz (yield from 1 lb)	1,152
4 oz	424
1 cup, chopped	524
1 cup, ground	411

Fresh, lean only
baked, with bone and skin
6.8 oz (yield from 1 lb)	421

baked, without bone and skin
8.1 oz (yield from 1 lb with fat)	495
4 oz	246
1 cup, chopped	304
1 cup, ground	239

Light-cured, lean with fat
raw, with bone and skin, 1 lb	1,100

baked, with bone and skin
11.3 oz (yield from 1 lb)	925
raw, without bone and skin, 1 lb	1,279

baked, without bone and skin
13.1 oz (yield from 1 lb)	1,075
4 oz	328
1 cup, chopped	405
1 cup, ground	318

Light-cured, lean only
baked, with bone and skin
8.7 oz (yield from 1 lb with fat)	460

baked, without bone and skin
    10.2 oz (yield from 1 lb with fat)   539
baked, without bone and skin
    4 oz   328
    1 cup, chopped   405
    1 cup, ground   318
Long-cured, dry, unbaked
    medium-fat, lean with fat, with bone and skin,
    4 oz   384
    lean, lean with fat, with bone and skin, 4 oz 302
Ham, minced, 4 oz   259

Pork, fresh

Boston butt, shoulder, with bone and skin, lean with fat
    raw, 1 lb   1,220
    roasted, 10.2 oz (yield from 1 lb)   1,024
Boston butt, shoulder, without bone and skin, lean with fat
    raw, 1 lb   1,302
    roasted
        10.9 oz (yield from 1 lb)   1,087
        1 cup, chopped   494
        1 cup, ground   388
Boston butt, shoulder, with bone and skin, lean only
    roasted, 8.1 oz (yield from 1 lb with fat)   559

Boston butt, shoulder, without bone and skin, lean only
  roasted

8.6 oz (yield from 1 lb with fat)	595
1 cup, chopped	342
1 cup, ground	268

Loin chops, with bone, lean with fat
  raw, 1 lb   1,065
  broiled

8.2 oz (yield from 1 lb)	911
1 chop, 2.7 oz	305
1 chop, 2 oz	227

Loin chops without bone, lean with fat
  raw, 1 lb   1,352
  broiled

10.4 oz (yield from 1 lb)	1,153
4 oz	411

Loin chops, with bone, lean only
  broiled

5.9 oz (yield from 1 lb with fat)	454
1 chop, 2 oz	151
1 chop, 1.5 oz	113

Loin chops, without bone, lean with fat

raw, 1 lb	1,065
baked or roasted, 8.6 oz (yield from 1 lb)	883

Loin roast, without bone, lean with fat
  raw, 1 lb   1,352
  baked or roasted

10.9 oz (yield from 1 lb)	1,115
4 oz	411
1 cup, chopped	507

Loin roast, with bone, lean only
baked or roasted
  6.9 oz (yield from 1 lb with fat)   495
  1 cup, chopped   356
Loin roast, without bone, lean only
baked or roasted
  8.7 oz (yield from 1 lb with fat)   627
  4 oz   288
  1 cup, chopped   356
Picnic, shoulder, with bone and skin, lean with fat
raw, 1 lb   1,083
simmered, 8.4. oz (yield from 1 lb)   890
Picnic, shoulder, without bone and skin, lean with fat
raw, 1 lb   1,315
simmered
  10.2 oz (yield from 1 lb)   1,085
  4 oz   424
  1 cup, chopped   524
Picnic, shoulder, with bone and skin, lean only
simmered, 6.2 oz (yield from 1 lb with fat) 373
Picnic, shoulder, without bone and skin, lean only
simmered
  7.6 oz (yield from 1 lb with fat)   456
  4 oz   241
  1 cup, chopped   297
Spareribs, with bone, lean with fat
raw, 1 lb   976
braised
  6.3 oz (yield from 1 lb)   792
  4 oz   499

Pork, specialty cuts, hog

Hearts

raw, 4 oz	128
braised, 4 oz	221
braised, 1 cup	283
Kidneys, raw, 8 oz	240
Liver	
raw, 1 lb	594
fried, 4 oz	205
Pancreas (Sweetbreads), 4 oz	274
Spleen, raw, 4 oz	122
Tongue, 4 oz	
raw, trimmed	244
braised	287

Pork, specialty cuts, pig, 4 oz

Feet, pickled	227
Salt Pork	
with skin	1,137
without skin	888
Stomach, scalded	274

7

Pork, cured, retail shoulder cuts (for other cured cuts see Bacon and Ham)

Boston butt, with bone and skin, lean with fat
unbaked, 1 lb	1,277
baked or roasted, 11 oz (yield from 1 lb)	1,030

Boston butt, without bone and skin, lean with fat
unbaked, 1 lb	1,320
baked or roasted	
11.8 oz from 1 lb	1,109
4 oz	374
1 cup, chopped	462
1 cup, ground	363

Boston butt, with bone and skin, lean only
baked or roasted, 9.1 oz (yield from 1 lb with fat)	629

Boston butt without bone and skin, lean only
baked or roasted	
9.8 oz (yield from 1 lb with fat)	678
4 oz	276
1 cup, chopped	340
1 cup, ground	267

Picnic, with bone and skin, lean with fat
unbaked, 1 lb	1,060
baked or roasted, 9.7 oz (yield from 1 lb)	888

Picnic, without bone and skin, lean with fat
unbaked, 1 lb	1,293
baked or roasted	
11.8 oz (yield from 1 lb)	1,085
4 oz	366
1 cup, chopped	452

1 cup, ground	355
Picnic, with bone and skin, lean only	
baked or roasted, 6.8 oz (yield from 1 lb with fat)	405
Picnic, without bone and skin, lean only	
baked or roasted	
8.3 oz (yield from 1 lb with fat)	496
4 oz	239
1 cup, chopped	295
1 cup, ground	232
Bacon, Canadian	
uncooked, 1 lb	980
fried, drained	
12 oz (approx. yield from 1 lb)	921
4 oz	311
1 slice 3⅜" wide	58
Bacon, cured	
raw, 1 lb	3,016
fried, drained	
5.1 oz (approx. yield from 1 lb)	860
1 thick slice	72
1 medium slice	43
1 thin slice	30

Veal, fresh, retail cuts

Chuck cuts and boneless for stew, lean with fat	
raw, with bone, 1 lb	628
stewed, with bone, 8.4 oz (yield from 1 lb)	564

raw, without bone, 1 lb	785
stewed, without bone	
10.6 oz (yield from 1 lb)	703
4 oz	267
1 cup, chopped	329

Loin cuts, lean with fat

raw, with bone, 1 lb	681
braised, or broiled, with bone	
9.5 oz (yield from 1 lb)	629
raw, without bone, 1 lb	821
braised or broiled, without bone	
11.4 oz (yield from 1 lb)	758
4 oz	245
1 cup, chopped	328

Plate (breast of veal), lean with fat

raw, with bone, 1 lb	828
braised or stewed, with bone,	
8.3 oz (yield from 1 lb)	718
raw, without bone, 1 lb	1,048
braised or stewed, without bone	
10.6 oz (yield from 1 lb)	906
4 oz	344

Rib roast, lean with fat

raw, with bone, 1 lb	723
roasted, with bone, 8.5 oz (yield from 1 lb)	648
raw, without bone, 1 lb	939
roasted, without bone	
11 oz (yield from 1 lb)	842
4 oz	305
1 cup, chopped	377

1 cup, ground	296
Round with rump (roasts and leg cutlets), lean with fat	
raw, with bone, 1 lb	573
braised or broiled, with bone	
8.7 oz (yield from 1 lb)	534
raw, without bone, 1 lb	744
braised or broiled, without bone	
11.3 oz (yield from 1 lb)	693
4 oz	245
1 cup, chopped	302

Veal, specialty cuts

Calf hearts	
raw, 4 oz	140
braised, 4 oz	236
1 cup	302
Calf kidneys, raw, 8 oz	256
Calves' liver	
raw, 4 oz	212
fried, 4 oz	296
Calf pancreas, 4 oz, raw	183
Calf tongue, 4 oz	
raw, trimmed	143
braised	181
Calf sweetbreads (thymus), 4 oz	
raw	106
braised	192

7

Cold Cuts, Sausages and other meats

Beaver, roasted, 8 oz.	563
Bockwurst	
1 lb (approx 7 links)	1,198
1 link (approx 2.3 oz)	172
Bologna	
without binders	
chub, 1 slice (3″ x ⅛″)	36
ring, 12 oz ring (15″ x 1⅜″)	942
sliced, 1 slice (approx 1 oz)	79
with cereal	
chub, 1 slice	34
ring, 12 oz ring	891
sliced, 1 slice	74
Brains, all types, fresh, raw, 8 oz	284
Capicola	
1 oz	141
1 slice	105
Cervelat, dry	
1 oz	128
4 slices	54
Frankfurter's without binders	
1 lb	1,343
1 frank (5″ x ¾″)	133
Frog's legs, raw	
whole, with bone, 1 lb	215
meat only, 4 oz	83
Meat Loaf, 4 oz	227

Muskrat, roasted, 4 oz	174
Rabbit, domesticated	
raw, whole, ready to cook, 1 lb	581
raw, meat only, 4 oz	184
stewed	
whole 8.6 oz (yield from 1 lb)	529
meat only	
4 oz	245
1 cup, chopped	302
1 cup, ground	238
Rabbit, wild	
whole, ready to cook, 1 lb	490
meat only, 4 oz	153
Raccoon, roasted, meat only, 4 oz	290
Reindeer, raw, lean meat only, 4 oz	144
Salami	
dry roll	
8¼ oz roll	1,053
1 slice	23
dry slice	
4 oz	509
1 slice	45
cooked	
8 oz	706
1 slice approx 1 oz	88
Sausage	
Blood pudding	
4 oz	447
1 slice	32

Polish
   4 oz   345

pork, raw
   2 oz patty   284
   1 oz link (4" x ⅞")   141

pork, cooked
   4 oz   543
   1 patty   129
   1 link   62

scrapple
   4 oz   244
   1 slice (⁹⁄₁₀ oz)   54

souse
   4 oz   205
   1 slice (1 oz)   51

Sheep tongue
   raw, trimmed, 8 oz   602
   braised, 4 oz   366

Snails, raw, 4 oz
   meat only   103
   Giant African, meat only   83

Spleen, all types, 4 oz   125

Terrapin (diamondback), raw
   in shell, 1 lb   106
   meat only, 4 oz   126

Thuringer cervelat (summer sausage)
   8 oz   697
   1 slice (approx 1 oz)   87

Turtle, green, raw
   in shell, 1 lb   97

meat only, 4 oz	101
Venison, raw, lean meat only, 4 oz	143

MEAT, COMMERCIALLY PACKAGED

Cured and processed meat, 1 oz unless noted

Bacon, cooked, 1 slice
  Hormel
    Black Label   35
    Range Label   45
    Red Label   37
  Oscar Mayer   40
  Swift   40
Bacon bits
  Wilson   140
Beef, chopped
  Eckrich, 1 slice   40
  Wilson   91
Beef, corned
  Dinty Moore   65
  Libby's   101
  Safeway   35

Beef, corned brisket
Swift	80
Wilson	45

Beef, dried
Swift	42

Beef, roast
Wilson	33

Beef, smoked
Safeway	35
spicy	40

Beef steaks
Hormel	92

Bologna, 1 slice
Eckrich	90
thick-sliced	160
Hormel	95
Swift	87
Wilson	87

Beef bologna
Eckrich	95
Beef Smorgas	70
Oscar Mayer	70

Coarse ground bologna
Hormel	75

Fine ground bologna
Hormel	80

Garlic bologna
Eckrich	95

Braunschweiger
Oscar Mayer	100

Wilson	90

Frankfurters, 1 frank

Eckrich	120
Jumbo	190
Skinless	150
Hormel	180
Wieners	105
Oscar Mayer	140
Wilson	140

Beef frankfurters, 1 frank

Eckrich	150
Jumbo	190
Hormel	
Wieners	105
Wranglers	160
Oscar Mayer	140
Vienna	130
Wilson	136

Ham, lunch meat

cooked

Eckrich, 1 slice	40
Hormel	35
Safeway	50
Oscar Mayer, 1 slice	30

chopped

Hormel	70
Oscar Mayer, 1 slice	65

chopped, smoked

Eckrich	40

Ham, whole, canned, 1 oz
Amber   110
Oscar Mayer   32
Swift   63
Wilson
  boned and rolled   56
  fully cooked   48
  Tender Made   44
Ham, whole, packaged, 1 oz
Hormel
  bone-in   52
  Cure 82   48
  Curemaster   35
Oscar Mayer   36
Swift   43
Wilson   48
Ham steaks, 1 slice
Oscar Mayer   70
Ham patties, 1 patty
Hormel   200
Swift   250
Ham and Cheese Loaf, 1 slice
Oscar Mayer   75
Honey Loaf, 1 slice
Eckrich   45
Oscar Mayer   40
Liver, beef
Swift   54
Liver cheese, 1 slice
Oscar Mayer   110

7

Old Fashioned Loaf, 1 slice
  Eckrich   75
  Oscar Mayer   65
Olive Loaf, 1 slice
  Oscar Mayer   65
Pastrami, 1 slice
  Eckrich   47
  Safeway   40
Pepperoni
  Hormel   140
  Swift   150
Pickle Loaf, 1 slice
  Eckrich   85
  Oscar Mayer   65
Polish Sausage
  Eckrich   100
  Frito-Lay   73
  Hormel   80
Pork Butt
  Wilson   72
Pork Loin
  Eckrich   47
Pork Steaks
  Hormel   73
Salami
  Hormel   327
  Oscar Mayer, 1 slice   50
Sausage, beef
  Eckrich   95

Sausage, pork
  Hormel   95
  Wilson   135

Sausage links, 1 sausage
  Hormel
    Brown 'n Serve   78
    Little Sizzlers   67
    Midget Links   112
  Oscar Mayer   65
  Swift   75

Sausage links, smoked, 1 sausage
  Eckrich   190
    skinless   115
    Smok-Y-Links   75
  Hormel   92
  Oscar Mayer   140

Scrapple
  Oscar Mayer   45

Sizzlean
  Swift   50

Spam
  Hormel   85

Summer Sausage
  Swift   90

Thuringer
  Hormel   100

Tripe
  Libby's canned   35

7

Veal Steaks
Hormel 35
breaded 60
Vienna Sausage, 1 sausage
Hormel 52
Libby's 84
with barbecue sauce 76

Canned Meat Entrees, 1 can, various sizes

Beef with barbecue sauce
Morton House 240
Beef, corned with cabbage
Hormel 150
Beef Goulash
Hormel 240
Beef sliced with gravy
Morton House 190
Chili con carne
Hormel 340
Libby's 130
Morton House 340
Chili con carne with beans
A&P 440
Hormel 320
Libby's 180
Morton House 340
Swanson 310
Hash, beef with potatoes
Dinty Moore 270

7

Hash, corned beef

Ann Page	400
Armour Star	435
Bounty	405
Broadcast	480
Libby's	160
Morton House	480
Wilson	480

Hash, roast beef

Hormel	375

Meatballs in gravy

Chef Boy-Ar-Dee	315

Pork, sliced with gravy

Morton House	190

Salisbury Steak with mushroom gravy

Morton House	160

Sloppy Joe

Banquet	250
Gebhardt	280
Hormel	365
Libby's	
beef	163
pork	139

Stew, beef

Armour Star	200
B & M	163
Bounty	213
Dinty Moore	184
Heinz	253
Morton House	312

James River Smithfield	186
Libby's	78
Morton House	240
Swanson	190
Wilson	202

Stew, lamb
B & M	247

Stew, meatball
Chef Boy-Ar-Dee	218
Libby's	121
Morton House	290

Stew, Mulligan
Dinty Moore	240

Frozen Meat Entrees, 1 whole package, various sizes (see also pp 385-391, Frozen Dinners)

Beef
Banquet	
Cookin' Bag	124
Buffet Supper, 32 oz	782
Green Giant Boil-in-Bag	130
Seabrook Farms	263
Stouffer's	235
Swanson	190
Swanson Hungry-Man	330

Beef goulash
Seabrook Farms — 198

Beef Pot Pie
Banquet — 412
Swanson — 443

Beef Stroganoff
Stouffer's — 390

Green Pepper Steak
Stouffer's — 350

Meat Loaf
Banquet
Buffet Supper, 32 oz — 1,445
Cookin' Bag — 224
Man Pleaser — 916
Morton — 430
Swanson — 330

Noodles and Beef
Banquet Buffet Supper, 32 oz — 754

Salisbury Steak
Banquet — 873
Green Giant Boil-in-Bag — 390
Morton — 490
Stouffer's — 500
Swanson — 370
Swanson Hungry-Man — 640

Salisbury Steak with gravy
Banquet
Buffet Supper, 32 oz — 1,454
Cookin' Bag — 246

Green Giant Oven Bake	290
Sausage, cheese, and tomato pie	
Weight Watchers	390
Sloppy Joe	
Banquet Cookin' Bag	199
Green Giant Boil-in-Bag	160
Steak	
Weight Watchers	390
Stew, Beef	
Banquet Buffet Supper, 32 oz	700
Green Giant Boil-in-Bag	160
Lambrecht	432
Seabrook Farms	229
Stouffer's	310
Stuffed Cabbage with beef	
Green Giant Oven Bake	220
Stuffed Green Pepper with Beef	
Green Giant Oven Bake	200

Meat Substitutes, 1 piece or slice

Morningstar Farms

Breakfast Links	62
Breakfast Patties	111
Breakfast Strips	38

Loma Linda

Bologna	190
Burgers	
Redi-Burger	150
Sizzle Burger	180
Frankfurters	110
Linketts	70
Little Links	45
Meatballs	48
Peanut Butter	
Nuteena	210
Proteena	160
Roast Beef	200
Salami	210
Sausage	
Breakfast Links	50
Breakfast Sausage	140
Swiss Steak	140
Tender Bits	20
Tender Rounds	50
Turkey	190
Vegeburger, 1 cup	240
Vegelona	160

POULTRY, FRESH

Chickens, fresh

Broilers
  broiled, with skin, giblets

7.1 oz (yield from 1 lb)	273
meat only, 4 oz	154
Capon, raw, ready to cook, 1 lb	382

Fryers

raw, ready to cook, 1 lb	382
fried, with skin, giblets	
8 oz (yield from 1 lb)	565
fried, without skin	
dark meat, 4 oz	249
light meat, 4 oz	223
1 back (approx 2 oz)	139
½ breast (approx 3.3 oz)	160
1 drumstick (approx 2 oz)	88
1 neck (approx 2 oz)	127
½ rib section (approx ¾ oz)	41
1 thigh (approx 2.3 oz)	122
1 wing (approx 1.8 oz)	82
skin only (approx 1 oz)	119

Roasters

raw, ready to cook, 1 lb	791
roasted, with skin, giblets	
8.4 oz (yield from 1 lb)	576

roasted, without skin, dark meat

4 oz	204
1 cup, chopped	258
1 cup, ground	202

roasted, without skin, light meat

4 oz	207
1 cup, chopped	255
1 cup, ground	200

Stewing hens or cocks

raw, ready to cook, 1 lb	987
stewed, with skin, giblets, 8 oz (yield from 1 lb)	708

stewed, without skin, dark meat

4 oz	235
1 cup, chopped	290
1 cup, ground	228

stewed, without skin, light meat

4 oz	204
1 cup, chopped	252
1 cup, ground	198

Chicken gizzards

raw, 1 lb	513

simmered

12 oz (yield from 1 lb)	497
4 oz	168
1 cup, chopped	215

Chicken hearts

raw, 4 oz	152

simmered

4 oz	221
1 cup, chopped	283

Chicken liver

raw, 1 lb	585
simmered	
4 oz	187
1 cup, chopped	231
1 liver 2″ x 2″ x ½″	45

Duck, fresh

Domesticated

raw, meat only, 4 oz	188
roasted, meat only, 4 oz	352

Wild

raw, meat only, 4 oz	157

Goose, fresh, domesticated

raw, whole, ready to cook, 1 lb	1,172
roasted	
whole, 8½ oz (yield from 1 lb)	1,022
meat only, 4 oz	266
meat and skin, 4 oz	503
Goose gizzards, raw, 1 lb	631
Goose liver, raw, 1 lb	826

7

Pheasant, fresh

raw, ready to cook, whole, 1 lb	596
raw, meat only, 4 oz	184

Quail, fresh, raw

whole, ready to cook, 1 lb	686
meat and skin only, 4 oz	196
giblets, 2 oz	100

Squab (Pigeon), fresh, raw

whole, dressed, 1 lb	569
meat only, 4 oz	162
light meat only, 4 oz	143

Turkey, fresh

raw, whole, ready to cook, 1 lb	722
roasted, whole, with giblets and skin 8.6 oz (yield from 1 lb)	644
roasted, dark meat without skin 4 oz	230

1 cup, chopped	284
1 cup, ground	223
roasted, light meat without skin	
4 oz	200
1 cup, chopped	246
1 cup, ground	194
roasted, skin only, 1 oz	256
giblets	
raw, 4 oz	170
simmered	
4 oz	254
1 cup, chopped	338
gizzards	
raw, 1 lb	712
simmered	
12 oz (yield from 1 lb)	659
4 oz	222
1 cup, chopped	284
hearts	
raw, 4 oz	169
simmered	
4 oz	245
1 cup, chopped	313
liver	
raw, 1 lb	626
simmered	
4 oz	197
1 cup, chopped	244

7

POULTRY, COMMERCIALLY CANNED, FROZEN, OR PACKAGED: 1 package, various sizes, unless noted (see also pp 385-391, Frozen Dinners)

Chicken

a la King
Banquet	138
Green Giant	170
Lambrecht	585
Stouffer's	330
Swanson	190

Boned
Hormel	110
Richardson & Robbins	328
Swanson	110

Chopped, 1 slice
Eckrich	47

Cacciatore
Seabrook Farms	248

Creamed
Stouffer's	300

Creole
  Weight Watchers — 250
Croquette
  Howard Johnson's — 505
Divan
  Stouffer's — 335
and Dumplings
  Banquet — 282
  Morton House, 8 oz — 363
  Swanson — 230
Escalloped
  Stouffer's — 500
Fricasse, 1 cup
  College Inn — 240
  Richardson & Robbins — 229
Fried
  Banquet — 259
  Morton — 600
  Swanson — 290
Livers with broccoli
  Weight Watchers — 220
with Noodles
  Banquet — 764
  Green Giant — 250
  Howard Johnson — 384
  Heinz — 186
Pot Pie
  Banquet — 412
  Morton — 318
  Stouffer's — 545

7

Swanson	430
Swanson Hungry-Man	770

with Rice

Morton House, 8 oz	460

Smoked

Safeway, 1 oz	50

Stew, 8 oz

B & M	168
Bounty	221
Libby's	88
Swanson, 7½ oz	180

White meat with peas and onions

Weight Watchers	270

Turkey

Boned

Hormel	90

with Giblet gravy

Banquet	128
Banquet Buffet Supper	170

Pot Pie

Banquet	415
Morton	390
Stouffer's	460
Swanson	430
Swanson Hungry-Man	770

7

Slices
Banquet	98
Banquet Buffet Supper	564
Green Giant	100
Morton Country Table	390
Morton House canned	140
Swanson	260
Swanson Hungry-Man	380

Tetrazzini
Stouffer's	480

Smoked
Eckrich, 1 slice	47
Safeway, 1 oz	50

SEAFOOD, FRESH,
4 oz unless noted

Abalone, raw	
in shell	47
meat only	111
Barracuda, Pacific, raw	
meat only	129
Bass, black sea, raw	
whole	41
meat only	106

7

Bass, all varieties, raw
whole	51
meat only	120

Blackfish, see Tautug

Bonito, raw
meat only	192

Butterfish, raw, meat only
gulf	108
northern	192

Catfish, raw, fillets 117

Caviar, sturgeon
granular
1 oz	74
1 Tbsp	42

pressed
1 oz	90
1 Tbsp	54

Clams, raw, meat only
hard or round
1 pt	363
8 oz	182
4 cherrystones or 5 littlenecks	56

soft
1 pt	372
8 oz	186

Cod
raw, fillets, 8 oz	176

broiled, with butter
1 steak	352

4 oz	192
dehydrated, lightly salted	308
1 cup, shredded	158
dried, salted	148
Crab, steamed, 8 oz	
in shell	100
meat only	211
Crab, deviled	
8 oz	427
Crab, Imperial	
8 oz	334
Crayfish, raw	
in shell	10
meat only	82
Croaker, Atlantic	
raw, meat only	109
Croaker, white	
raw, meat only	95
Croaker, yellow	
raw, meat only	101
Cusk	
raw, meat only	85
steamed, meat only	120
Eulachon, see Smelt	
Finnan Haddie	
meat only	117
Flounder, fillets	
raw	89
baked with butter	229

Grouper, raw

whole	42
meat only	99

Haddock

raw

whole, 1 lb	172
fillets, 1 lb	360
fried, breaded, 4 oz	187

Halibut, Atlantic or Pacific

raw

whole, 1 lb	268
fillets, 1 lb	452
broiled with butter, fillets, 4 oz	199

Herring

Atlantic, raw

whole, 1 lb	405
meat only, 4 oz	200

Pacific

raw, meat only, 4 oz	111
salted (in brine), 4 oz	247

smoked, 4 oz

bloaters	222
hard	340
kippers	239

Inconnu, raw

whole	104
meat only	166

Kingfish, raw

whole	52

meat only	119
Lake Herring (Cisco), raw	
whole	55
meat only	110
Lake Trout, raw	
whole	70
meat only	190
Ling Cod, raw	
whole	44
meat only	96
Lobster, northern	
in shell, 1 lb	
raw	107
cooked	112
Mackerel, Atlantic	
raw, 1 lb	
whole	468
fillets	866
broiled with butter, fillets,	
13 oz yield from 1 lb	861
4 oz	268
Mackerel, Pacific, raw	
whole	130
meat only	181
Mackerel, salted	345
Mackerel, smoked	248
Mullet, raw	
whole	88
meat only	166

Muskellunge, raw
whole	60
meat only	124

Mussels, Atlantic or Pacific, raw
in shell	38
meat only	108

Ocean Perch, Atlantic
raw
whole	31
meat only	100
fried, breaded	258

Ocean Perch, Pacific, raw
whole	29
meat only	108

Octopus, raw   83

Oysters, raw
Eastern
in shell, 1 lb	30
meat only, 4 oz	75
1 medium	20

Pacific Western
meat only, 4 oz	105
1 medium	55

Oysters, cooked
fried, breaded, 1 medium	25

Pickerel, raw   95

Perch, raw
white
whole	48
meat only	134

yellow
   whole   40
   meat only   103

Pike, raw
  blue
   whole   45
   meat only   100
  northern
   whole   26
   meat only   100
  walleye
   whole   60
   meat only   105

Pompano, raw
  whole   106
  meat only   188

Porgy, raw   52
  meat only   127

Rockfish
  raw   110
  steamed   115

Roe, raw
  carp, cod, haddock, herring, pike, and shad   148
  salmon, sturgeon, and turbot   236

Sablefish, raw
  whole   90
  meat only   216

Salmon, raw
  Atlantic
   whole   160

meat only	246
King (Chinook) meat only	252
Salmon, smoked	200
Sand Dab, raw	
meat only	89
Sardines, Pacific	
raw, meat only	180
Sauger, raw	
whole	34
meat only	95
Scallops, meat only	
raw	92
steamed	127
Sea Bass, white	
raw, meat only	109
Shad, raw	
whole	92
meat only	192
Sheepshead, Atlantic, raw	
whole	60
meat only	128
Shrimp	
raw, whole	
in shell	72
shelled	100
fried, breaded	250
Skate	
raw, meat only	111
Smelt, raw	
whole	60

meat only	110
Snapper, Red and Gray, raw	
whole	55
meat only	106
Sole, raw	
whole	29
meat only (fillet)	90
Spanish Mackerel, raw	
whole	142
meat only	200
Spot	
raw, meat only	250
Squid	
raw, meat only	95
Sturgeon, meat only	
raw	105
steamed	180
Sturgeon, smoked	170
Sucker, carp	
raw	48
meat only	125
Sucker, white and mullet, raw	
whole	195
meat only	118
Swordfish, meat only	
raw	138
broiled in butter	185
Tautug (Blackfish), raw	
whole	37
meat only	101

Tilefish

raw

    whole   46

    meat only   90

baked, meat only   155

Tomcod, raw

whole   34

meat only   88

Trout, Brook, raw

whole   56

meat only   115

Trout, Rainbow, raw

meat only   220

Tuna, raw, meat only

bluefin   165

yellowfin   150

Turbot, Greenland, raw

whole   86

meat only   166

Weakfish

raw

    whole   66

    meat only   138

broiled in butter   230

Whitefish, raw

whole   82

meat only   177

smoked   177

Wreckfish

raw, meat only   130

Yellowtail
raw, meat only   157

SEAFOOD, CANNED
AND FROZEN

Catfish, ocean
Gorton's, 1 pkg   286
Clams
Doxsee
6 oz   84
8 oz   112
12 oz   147
Howard Johnson's
5 oz   395
Croquettes, 1 pkg   608
Mrs. Paul's 1 cake   180
Thins, 1 cake   155
Sticks, 1 stick   48
Sau-Sea, 1 jar   99
Snow's   60
Cod, 1 pkg
fillets
Gorton's   355
San Juan   336
Ship Ahoy   336

sticks

Bird's Eye	552
Gorton's	830

Crab

Gold Seal, 1 can	185
Icy Point, 1 can	215
Mrs. Paul's, 1 cake	60
Pillar Rock, 1 can	216
Ship Ahoy, 8 oz	210
Wakefield's, 6 oz	160

Crepes, 5½ oz

Mrs. Paul's

Clam	280
Crab	240
Scallop	220
Shrimp	250

Croquettes

Howard Johnson's

Shrimp with Newburg Sauce	480

Eel, smoked 185

Vita	402

Fish Au Gratin

Mrs. Paul's 1 pkg	250

Fish cakes, fillets and sticks, 1 piece

Mrs. Paul's	105
Beach Haven	110
Thins	160

Fish and Chips

Swanson, 1 pkg	290

Fish Parmesan
  Mrs. Paul's, 1 pkg | 220
Flounder
  Mrs. Paul's, 1 pkg | 110
  Weight Watchers, 1 pkg | 160
Gelfilte Fish, 1 oz
  Manischewitz | 23
  Mother's | 14
  Rokeach | 19
Haddock au Gratin
  Howard Johnson's | 315
Haddock fillets
  Gorton's, 1 pkg | 360
  Mrs. Paul's, 1 piece | 115
Haddock with stuffing
  Weight Watchers, 1 pkg | 180
Herring, pickled, 1 oz
  Vita | 40
Oysters, 1 cup
  Bumblebee | 172
Perch, fried, 1 piece
  Mrs. Paul's | 125
Perch, ocean with broccoli
  Weight Watchers, 1 pkg | 190
Salmon, canned, 1 can
  blueback
    Icy Point
      3¾-oz can | 181
      7¾-oz can | 376

Coho steak
  Icy Point
    3¾-oz can   162
pink
  Del Monte
    7¾-oz can   310
red
  Icy Point
    1-lb. can   775
  Pillar Rock
    3¾-oz can   181
    7¾-oz can   376
red sockeye
  Del Monte
    7¾-oz can   340
  Bumblebee
    1 cup   286
Sardines, 1 oz
  Del Monte   44
  Underwood
    in mustard sauce   52
    in soya bean oil   62
    in tomato sauce   330
Scallops
  Mrs. Paul's, 3½ oz   210
Seafood combination
  Mrs. Paul's   510
Shrimp
  Bumblebee, 1 can   90

Icy Point, 1 can	148
Pillar Rock, 1 can	148
Mrs. Paul's, 1 oz	57
Sau-Sea, 1 oz	80
Shad Roe	
Bumblebee, 1 can	259
Shrimp and Scallops	
Stouffer's, 1 pkg	400
Sole	
Mrs. Paul's, 4½ oz	160
Ship Ahoy, 1 pkg	310
with peas, mushrooms, and lobster sauce	
Weight Watchers, 1 pkg	200
Tuna, canned in oil, drained	
Bumblebee, 1 cup	334
Chicken of the Sea	
3¼-oz can	224
6½-oz can	447
9¼-oz can	636
12½-oz can	860
Del Monte, 6½-oz can	450
Gold Seal, 5-oz can	278
Icy Point, 5-oz can	278
Pillar Rock, 5-oz can	278
Snow Mist, 5-oz can	278
Van Camp, 6¼-oz can	440
Tuna, canned, solid, in water	
Bumblebee, 1 cup	300
Chicken of the Sea, 7-oz can	216

Tuna, creamed, with peas
Green Giant Boil-in-Bag   140
Tuna Pot Pies
Banquet   478
Morton   385
Star Kist   397
Turbot with peas and carrots
Weight Watchers, 1 pkg   280

CHAPTER 8

Fruits and Vegetables

FRESH FRUITS AND VEGETABLES

Acerolas (West Indian Cherries)
    whole, 1 lb   104
    pitted, 4 oz   32
    3 cherries   7
Amaranth
    whole, 1 lb   100
    leaves only, 1 lb   160
Apples
    with skin
        1 lb   242

1 apple (3¼", 2 per lb)	123
1 apple (2¾", 3 per lb)	80
1 apple (2½", 4 per lb)	61
chopped, 1 cup	73
pared	
1 apple (3¼", 2 per lb)	107
1 apple (2¾", 3 per lb)	70
1 apple (2½", 4 per lb)	53
chopped, 1 cup	68

Apples, dehydrated

uncooked	
8 oz	800
1 cup	355
cooked, sweetened	
8 oz	175
1 cup	195

Apples, dried

uncooked	
8 oz	625
1 cup	234
cooked, unsweetened	
8 oz	177
1 cup	199
cooked, sweetened	
8 oz	254
1 cup	314

Apricots

whole	
1 lb	217
1 apricot	18

pitted, halves
1 lb	231
1 cup	79

Apricots, dehydrated
uncooked
8 oz	755
1 cup	330

cooked, sweetened
8 oz	271
1 cup	339

Apricots, dried
uncooked
8 oz	590
1 cup	340
10 medium halves	90

cooked, unsweetened, with liquid
8 oz	195
1 cup	210
cooked, sweetened, 1 cup	329

Artichokes
raw, whole, 1 lb	85
boiled, drained, 1 whole bud	67

Asparagus
raw
whole, 1 lb	66
cuts, 1 cup	35

boiled, drained
1 medium spear	3
cuts, 1 cup	29

Avocados, California

whole, 1 lb	589
peeled and pitted, 1 average	370
diced, 1 cup	260
mashed, 1 cup	390

Avocados, Florida

whole, 1 lb	389
peeled and pitted, 1 average	200
diced, 1 cup	190
mashed, 1 cup	300

Bamboo shoots, raw

8 oz	61
1 cup, cuts	40

Bananas

whole

1 large (10″)	119
1 medium (9″)	103
1 small (8″)	83

1 cup

sliced	135
mashed	190

Bananas, dehydrated

flakes, 1 cup	340

Bananas, red

whole, 1 average (7¼″)	118
sliced, 1 cup	135

Bean Sprouts, mung

uncooked

8 oz	80
1 cup	37

boiled, drained
  8 oz   65
  1 cup   35

Bean sprouts, soy
uncooked
  8 oz   105
  1 cup   48
boiled, drained
  8 oz   86
  1 cup   48

Beet greens
raw, trimmed, 1 lb   61
boiled, drained
  8 oz   41
  1 cup   26

Beets
raw, trimmed
  1 lb   137
  whole, 1 beet (2″) 21
  diced, 1 cup   58
boiled, drained
  whole, 1 beet   16
  diced, 1 cup   58
  sliced, 1 cup   66

Blackberries
1 lb   250
1 cup   84

Blueberries
1 lb   260
1 cup   90

8

Broccoli
raw
whole, 1 lb	90
trimmed, 1 lb	145

boiled, drained
8 oz	59
1 average stalk 6½ oz	47
cuts, 1 cup	40

Brussel Sprouts
raw
whole, 1 lb	200
trimmed, 1 lb	190

boiled, drained
8 oz	82
1 cup	55
1 average sprout	7

Cabbage, Chinese (Celery Cabbage), raw
whole, 1 lb	62
trimmed, 1 lb	65
cuts, 1 cup	11
strips, 1 cup	8

Cabbage, green
raw
whole, 1 lb	98
trimmed, 1 lb	110
chopped, 1 cup	22
sliced, 1 cup	17
ground, 1 cup	36
boiled, drained, 1 cup	30

Cabbage, dehydrated, 1 oz
87

Cabbage, red, raw
  whole, 1 lb   127
  trimmed, 1 lb   141
  sliced, 1 cup   22
Cabbage, savoy, raw
  whole, 1 lb   98
  trimmed, 1 lb   109
  sliced, 1 cup   17
Cabbage, spoon (Bakchoy)
  raw
    whole, 1 lb   73
    trimmed, 1 lb   70
    cuts, 1 cup   11
  boiled, drained, cuts, 1 cup   24
Cantaloupe
  one 5-inch melon   95
  cubed, 1 cup   48
Carambola, raw
  whole, 1 lb   150
  peeled and seeded, 8 oz   80
Carissas (Natal plums), raw
  whole, 1 lb   273
  peeled and seeded, 8 oz   155
  sliced, 1 cup   105
Carrot
  raw
    whole, 1 lb   156
    whole scraped
      8 oz   95
      1 medium   21

diced, 1 cup	60
slices, 1 cup	53
boiled, drained, 1 cup	45
Carrot, dehydrated, 1 oz	100
Casaba melon	
whole	61
cubed, 1 cup	45
Cauliflower	
raw	
whole, 1 lb	48
flowerets	
1 lb	120
1 cup	27
chopped, 1 cup	30
boiled, drained, 1 cup	29
Celeriac root, raw	
whole, 1 lb	155
pared, 1 root approx 1 oz	11
Celery	
raw	
whole, 1 lb	58
1 large outer stalk (8″)	7
1 small inner stalk (5″)	3
chopped, 1 cup	20
boiled, drained, 1 cup	22
Chard, Swiss	
raw	
whole, 1 lb	113
1 lb, then trimmed	104

boiled, drained
  leaves and stalks, 1 cup — 26
  leaves only, 1 cup — 32

Chayote
  raw, 1 medium squash — 56

Cherimoya, raw
  whole, 1 lb — 247
  peeled and seeded, 8 oz — 215

Cherries
  sour, red
    whole
      1 lb — 213
      1 cup — 60
    pitted, 1 cup — 90
  sweet
    whole
      1 lb — 286
      1 cup — 82
    pitted
      1 cup — 102
      1 average cherry — 5

Chervil
  raw, 1 oz — 16

Chives, raw
  whole, 1 lb — 128
  chopped, 1 Tbsp — 1

Coconut, raw
  in shell, 1 coconut (4½″ and 27 oz) — 1,375
  shelled, meat only, 4 oz — 392

shredded, 1 cup

loosely packed	277
firmly packed	450

Coconut, dried, shredded

unsweetened

4 oz	750
1 cup	622

sweetened

4 oz	622
1 cup	515

Collards

raw

whole, 1 lb	180
leaves only, 1 lb	205

boiled

leaves only	60
with stems, 1 cup	43

Corn, sweet

raw, on the cob, 1 lb	240

boiled, drained

on the cob, 1 ear (5″)	70
kernels, 1 cup	140

Corn Salad, raw

whole, 1 lb	90
trimmed, 1 lb	95

Crab apples, raw

whole, 1 lb	280
trimmed	309

Cranberries

whole, 1 lb	200

without stems, 1 cup	52
chopped, 1 cup	50
Cranberries, dehydrated, 1 oz	100
Cucumber	
1 lb	65
1 average (7½″)	35
sliced, 1 cup	15
Currants	
black	
whole, 1 lb	240
trimmed, 1 cup	60
red or white	
whole, 1 lb	220
trimmed, 1 cup	55
Dandelion greens	
raw, trimmed, 1 lb	205
boiled, drained, 1 cup	
loosely packed	35
firmly packed	70
Dates, domestic	
whole, 1 lb	1,081
pitted, 1 lb	1,243
chopped, 1 cup	488
1 average date	22
Dock (Sorrel)	
raw, whole, 1 lb	89
boiled, drained, 1 cup	38
Eggplant	
raw	
whole, 1 lb	92

diced, 1 cup	50
boiled, drained, 1 cup	38

Elderberries

whole, 1 lb	310
without stems, 8 oz	160

Endive (French or Belgian) bleached (Chicory)

trimmed, 1 lb	68
1 head (6″)	8
1 small leave	½
chopped, 1 cup	14

Escarole

whole, 1 lb	80
large outer leaf	5
small inner leaf	½
chopped, 1 cup	10

Fennel, raw

whole, 1 lb	120
trimmed, 2 oz	15

Figs, raw

whole, 1 lb	360
1 medium (2¼″)	40
dried	
8 oz	620
1 medium (2″)	58

Garlic, raw

whole, 2 oz	68
peeled	
2 oz	80
1 clove	3

Ginger root
whole, 1 lb ... 205
peeled, 1 oz ... 14
Green (Snap) Beans, 1 cup ... 31
Gooseberries
1 lb ... 177
1 cup ... 59
Grapefruit
pink
whole, 1 lb ... 89
sections, 1 cup ... 80
white
whole, 1 lb ... 86
sections, 1 cup ... 80
Grapes
American slipskin: Concord, Delaware, Niagara
whole, 1 lb ... 197
seeded
1 cup ... 70
1 grape ... 2
European close skin: Malaga, Muscat, Thompson
whole, 1 lb ... 270
seeded, 1 cup ... 100
seedless
1 cup ... 107
1 grape ... 3½
Ground-cherries, raw
whole, 1 lb ... 220
without husks
1 lb ... 240
1 cup ... 74
Guava
whole, 1 lb ... 275
trimmed, 8 oz ... 140
1 average ... 58
Honeydew Melon
whole, 1 lb ... 94
cubed, 1 cup ... 56

Jack Fruit

whole, 1 lb	125
peeled and seeded, 8 oz	110

Jujubes (Chinese dates)

fresh

whole, 1 lb	444
seeded, 8 oz	238

dried

whole, 1 lb	1,160
seeded, 8 oz	650

Kale

raw

whole, 1 lb	129
without stems, 1 lb	155
leaves only, 4 oz	80

boiled, drained

1 cup	31
leaves only, 1 cup	44

Kohlrabi

raw

whole, 1 lb	96
pared	
8 oz	65
diced, 1 cup	40
boiled, drained, 1 cup	40

Kumquats

whole, 1 lb	274
trimmed	
8 oz	150

8

1 medium	12
Leeks, raw	
whole, 1 lb	123
bulb and lower leaf	
8 oz	116
1 medium	17
Lettuce	
Boston	
whole	
1 lb	47
1 head (5″)	23
1 large, 2 medium or 3 small leaves	2
chopped, 1 cup	8
Iceberg	
whole	
1 lb	56
1 head (6″)	70
1 medium leaf	3
chopped, 1 cup	7
Loose Leaf	
whole	
1 lb	52
3 large leaves	15
chopped, 1 cup	10
Romaine or cos	
whole	
1 lb	52
1 leaf	2
chopped, 1 cup	10

8

Limes
  whole, 1 lb   106
  pulp only, 1 lime   19

Loganberries
  whole, 1 lb   267
  trimmed
    8 oz   140
    1 cup   90

Loqats
  whole, 1 lb   168
  seeded
    8 oz   110
    1 medium   6

Mangoes, whole
  1 lb   200
  1 medium   150
  1 cup   110

Mushrooms, raw
  whole, 1 lb   123
  chopped, 1 cup   20

Mustard Greens
  raw
    whole
      1 lb   57
      trimmed, 8 oz   70
  boiled, drained, leaves only
    8 oz   52
    1 cup   32

Mustard Spinach (Tendergreens)
  raw, whole, 1 lb   100

boiled, drained	
8 oz	37
1 cup	30
Nectarines, whole	
1 lb	267
1 medium	88
New Zealand Spinach	
raw, whole, 1 lb	86
boiled, drained	
8 oz	30
1 cup	23
Okra	
raw	
whole, 1 lb	140
trimmed, 8 oz	80
boiled, drained, sliced, 1 cup	45
Onions, mature	
raw	
whole, 1 lb	157
trimmed	
8 oz	85
1 medium	40
chopped, 1 cup	65
chopped, 1 Tbsp	4
grated, 1 cup	90
boiled, drained, 1 cup	60
Onions, young green	
whole, 1 lb	157
bulb and top	
trimmed, 1 lb	164

chopped, 1 cup	36
chopped, 1 Tbsp	2
top only, chopped	
1 cup	27
1 Tbsp	2

Onions, Welsh
raw

whole, 1 lb	100
trimmed, 8 oz	78

Oranges
whole

1 lb	162
1 medium	64
diced, 1 cup	103

Papaw
whole

1 lb	290
1 medium	83
peeled and seeded	
8 oz	185
1 cup	210

Papayas
whole

1 lb	120
1 medium	120
peeled and seeded	
8 oz	90
cubed, 1 cup	55

Parsley

whole, 1 lb	200
chopped	
1 cup	26
1 Tbsp	2
1 sprig	4

Parsnips

raw, whole, 1 lb	293
boiled, drained	
diced, 1 cup	100
mashed, 1 cup	140

Passion Fruit

whole	
1 lb	210
1 medium	15
shelled, 8 oz	200

Peaches

whole, 1 lb	150
peeled, 1 medium	38
pared, diced, 1 cup	70

Pears, 1 pear

Bartlett	200
Bosc	85
D'Anjou	120

Peas, green immature

raw	
whole, 1 lb	150
shelled	
1 lb	380
1 cup	120

boiled, drained

8 oz	160
1 cup	115

Peas, mature, dried
raw
whole

1 lb	1,540
1 cup	680
split, uncoated, 1 cup	700
cooked, split, uncoated, 1 cup	230

Pea Pods (Snow Peas)

whole, 1 lb	228

Pepper, Hot chili, green, raw

whole, 1 lb	120
seeded, 8 oz	85

Pepper, Hot chili, red
raw

whole, 1 lb	400
seeded, 8 oz	145
pods, dried, 1 Tbsp	25

Peppers, Sweet, green, raw
whole

1 lb	80
1 pepper, fancy grade large	35
1 pepper, No 1 grade	15
chopped, 1 cup	33

Peppers, Sweet, red, raw

whole, 1 lb	110
seeded and cored, 8 oz	70
chopped, 1 cup	47

8

Persimmon
  Japanese or Kaki
    whole, 1 lb   286
    seedless, 1 lb   295
    trimmed, 1 medium   130
  native
    whole
      1 lb   475
      1 medium   32
    trimmed and seeded, 8 oz   65

Pigeon peas
  raw, whole, 1 lb   210
  dried, 8 oz   760

Pineapple
  whole, 1 lb   125
  cubed, 1 cup   80

Pitanga (Surinam Cherries)
  whole
    1 lb   187
    4 medium   10
  pitted, 1 cup   87

Plantains, raw
  whole, 1 lb   390
  peeled, 8 oz   270
  1 banana (10″)   285

Plums
  Damson
    whole
      1 lb   272

1 medium	7
pitted, 8 oz	150
Japanese	
whole	
1 lb	205
1 medium	32
pitted, 8 oz	110
Prune type	
whole	
1 lb	320
1 medium	21
pitted, 8 oz	170
Poke Shoot (Pokeberry)	
raw, 1 lb	104
boiled, drained, 1 cup	33
Pomegranate	
whole	
1 lb	194
1 medium	100
Potatoes	
raw	
whole, 1 lb	280
peeled, 1 cup	114
baked in skin	
4 oz	81
1 long	145
boiled in skin	
4 oz	79
1 long	173
1 round	104

8

boiled, peeled
  4 oz   74
  1 cup   100
fried, 4 oz   275
hash brown, 4 oz   260
mashed, with milk and butter
  4 oz   107
  1 cup   137
scalloped, with cheese, 4 oz   118

Prickly Pears, raw
whole, 1 lb   84
peeled and seeded, 8 oz   96

Prunes, dehydrated, uncooked
8 oz   780
1 cup   344

Pumpkin, raw
whole, 1 lb   83
pulp only, 8 oz   60

Purslane leaves
raw, whole, 1 lb   95
boiled, drained, 1 cup   27

Quinces
whole, 1 lb   158
peeled and seeded, 8 oz   130

Radishes, raw
whole
  1 lb   49
  10 medium   8
sliced, 1 cup   20

Radishes, Oriental

whole, 1 lb	57
without tops, 1 lb	67
pared, 8 oz	45

Raisins, seedless

8 oz	655
1 cup loose	420
1 cup firmly packed	477

Raspberries

black

1 lb	330
1 cup	98

red

1 lb	260
1 cup	70

Rhubarb

raw

whole, 1 lb	33
trimmed, 1 lb	60
diced, 1 cup	20
cooked, sweetened, 1 cup	381

Rose Apples

whole, 1 lb	170
trimmed and seeded, 8 oz	138

Rutabagas

raw

whole, 1 lb	177
trimmed, 8 oz	105
diced, 1 cup	60

boiled, drained
  cubes, 1 cup   60
  mashed, 1 cup   84

Sapodillas
  whole, 1 lb   323
  peeled and seeded, 8 oz   202

Shallots, raw
  whole, 1 oz   18
  peeled
    1 oz   20
    1 Tbsp   7

Soursop, raw
  whole, 1 lb   200
  peeled and seeded, 8 oz   149

Soybean curd (Tofu)
  4 oz   82

Spinach
  raw
    whole, 1 lb   85
    trimmed
      leaves, 1 cup   9
      chopped, 1 cup   14
  boiled, drained, leaves, 1 cup   41

Squash, summer
  raw
    whole, 1 lb   85
    trimmed, 8 oz   25
    diced, 1 cup   35
  boiled, drained, 1 cup   30

Squash, winter

raw, whole, 1 lb	150
baked, 8 oz	120

Strawberries, whole

1 lb	161
trimmed, 1 lb	168
1 cup	55

Sugar Apples (Sweetsop)

whole, 1 lb	192
peeled and seeded	
8 oz	220
1 cup	235

Swamp Cabbage

raw	
whole, 1 lb	107
trimmed, 1 lb	132
boiled, drained, 8 oz	48

Sweet Potatoes

raw, whole, 1 lb	420
baked in skin, 4 oz	125

Tamarinds

whole, 1 lb	520
shelled and seeded, 8 oz	540

Tomatoes, green

whole, 1 lb	99

Tomatoes, ripe

raw	
whole	
1 lb	100
1 medium	25

8

sliced, 1 cup	40
boiled, 1 cup	63
Towel Gourd	
whole, 1 lb	70
pared, 8 oz	40
Turnip Greens	
raw	
whole, 1 lb	107
trimmed, 1 lb	127
boiled	
8 oz	46
1 cup	30
Turnips	
raw	
whole, 1 lb	117
cubed, 1 cup	39
boiled, drained	
8 oz	52
1 cup	36
mashed	53
Vinespinach (Basella), raw, 8 oz	44
Water Chestnuts, Chinese	
raw, whole, 1 lb	276
Watercress	
whole	
1 lb	80
1 cup	7
chopped, 1 cup	24
Watermelon	
whole, 1 lb	54

8

1 wedge (4" x 8")	110
diced, 1 cup	42
Wax (Yellow) Beans	
1 cup	29
Yam Beans, raw	
whole, 1 lb	225
pared, 8 oz	130
Yams, raw	
whole, 1 lb	395
pared, 4 oz	115
Zucchini (see Summer Squash)	

FRUIT, COMMERCIALLY PACKAGED, CANNED OR FROZEN,
½ cup unless noted

Apples and Apricots	
Mott's	104
Apples and Cherries	
Mott's	110
Apples and Pineapples	
Mott's	127

Apples and Raspberries
Mott's   105
Applesauce
Del Monte   85
Mott's   45
S & W   48
Stokely-Van Camp   90
Tillie Lewis   60
Town House   85
Apricots
Del Monte   100
Libby's   100
Stokely-Van Camp   110
Tillie Lewis   60
Town House   80
Blackberries
S & W   36
Blueberries
Seabrook Farms   45
Boysenberries
S & W   32
Cherries
Del Monte Light   95
   Dark   90
   Dark pitted   95
Libby's   100
S & W   50
Stokely-Van Camp   50
Cherries, maraschino
Vita 1 cherry   20

Cranberry and Orange
Ocean Spray 100
Cranberry Sauce
Ocean Spray 90
Currants
Del Monte 190
Dates
Bordo 330
Dromedary 397
Dromedary pitted 376
Figs
Del Monte 100
S & W, 6 figs 49
Fruit Cocktail
Del Monte 85
Dole 72
Libby's 75
S & W 35
Stokely-Van Camp 95
Tillie Lewis 50
Town House 85
Fruit Salad
Del Monte 85
Del Monte Tropical 100
Kraft 48
Libby's 90
S & W 35
Stokely-Van Camp 95
Fruits and Peels
Liberty 388

Grapefruit sections
Del Monte 45
Kraft 43
S & W 36
Tillie Lewis 45

Mixed Fruit
Birds Eye 105

Melon Balls
Birds Eye, 1 pkg 144

Oranges
Del Monte 75
Kraft 52
S & W 27

Peaches
Birds Eye 72
Del Monte 85
Highway 70
S & W 25
Scotch Buy 70
Seabrook Farms 105
Stokely-Van Camp 90
Town House, heavy syrup 95
Town House, extra heavy syrup 130

Peaches and Strawberries
Birds Eye 80

Pears
Del Monte 80
Libby's 85
Libby's Juice Pack 75
Highway 80

Scotch Buy 70
S & W 28
Stokely-Van Camp 105
Tillie Lewis 50

Pineapple
Del Monte in juice 70
Del Monte in syrup 95
Dole in juice 65
Dole in syrup 85
S & W 50
Town House in juice 75
Town House in syrup 95

Plums
Del Monte 95
Libby's 105
S & W 50
Stokely-Van Camp 120
Tillie Lewis 70

Prunes
Del Monte 115
Heart's Delight 210
Sunsweet 196

Raspberries
Birds Eye 120
Seabrook Farms 120

Rhubarb
Birds Eye 138

Strawberries
Birds Eye 90
Birds Eye slices 145

Seabrook Farms	42
Seabrook Farms slices	140
S & W	20

VEGETABLES, COMMERCIALLY PACKAGED, CANNED OR FROZEN,
1 cup unless noted

Artichoke Hearts

Birds Eye	53

Asparagus, cuts

Green Giant	40
Kounty Kist	40
Lindy	39
Stokely-Van Camp	44

Asparagus, Spears

Del Monte	35
Green Giant	40
Le Sueur	38
S & W	18
Town House	35

Asparagus, frozen

Birds Eye	61
with Hollandaise Sauce, 1 pkg	290

Green Giant	90
Seabrook Farms	46
Bamboo Shoots	
Chun King	30
La Choy	23
Bean Sprouts	
Chun King	40
La Choy	24
Beets, cut	
Del Monte	70
Libby's	70
Stokely-Van Camp	90
Beets, diced	
Comstock	82
Libby's	70
Stokely-Van Camp	70
Beets, Harvard	
Greenwood	104
Libby's	160
Lord Mott	80
Stokely-Van Camp	160
Beets, pickled	
Del Monte	150
Greenwood	150
Libby's	150
Lord Mott	150
Stokely-Van Camp	190
Town House	145
Beets, sliced	
Del Monte	70

8

Libby's	70
Lord Mott	50
S & W	56
Stokely-Van Camp	80
Beets, whole	
Del Monte	70
Libby's	70
Stokely-Van Camp	85
Beets, frozen	
Birds Eye	105
Broccoli, frozen	
Birds Eye	25
with cheese	110
in hollandaise	200
Green Giant	30
in butter	90
in cheese sauce	130
with cauliflower and carrots	140
Kounty Kist	30
Seabrook Farms	46
Stouffer's Au gratin	340
Brussels Sprouts	
Birds Eye	30
Green Giant	50
in butter sauce	110
in cheese sauce	170
Kounty Kist	50
Seabrook Farms	76
Cabbage	
Greenwood	150

Lord Mott	120
Carrots, diced	
Comstock	48
Del Monte	61
Libby's	40
S & W	44
Stokely-Van Camp	60
Carrots, sliced	
Birds Eye, in buttersauce	340
in sugar	194
Comstock	35
Del Monte	58
Green Giant, in butter sauce	100
Libby's	42
Lord Mott	50
Stokely-Van Camp	50
Cauliflower	
Birds Eye	61
with cheese sauce	130
Green Giant	30
with cheese sauce	130
Kounty Kist	26
Seabrook Farms	26
Collard Greens	
Birds Eye	30
Seabrook Farms	44
Corn, Yellow, canned	
cream style	
Birds Eye	170
Del Monte	210

Green Giant	210
S & W	168
Stokely-Van Camp	210
liquid pack	
Del Monte	170
Green Giant	160
Kounty Kist	180
Le Sueur	170
Libby's	160
S & W	104
Stokely-Van Camp	180
vacuum pack	
Del Monte	200
Green Giant	160
Kounty Kist	160
Stokely-Van Camp	240
with peppers	
Del Monte	190
Green Giant	150
Corn, Yellow, frozen	
Birds Eye in butter sauce	200
Green Giant in butter sauce	190
with peppers	180
Stouffer's, 1 pkg	465
Corn, White, frozen and canned	
Birds Eye creamed	170
with peas	140
Del Monte creamed	190
kernels	150
Green Giant	130

Kounty Kist	140
Eggplant Parmesan	
Mrs. Paul's	364
Eggplant slices	
Mrs. Paul's	613
Eggplant sticks	
Mrs. Paul's	254
Kale	
Seabrook Farms	60
Mixed Vegetables, canned	
Del Monte	79
La Choy	35
Libby's	78
Stokely-Van Camp	81
Town House	88
Mixed Vegetables, frozen	
Birds Eye	145
Chun King	23
Green Giant	90
Kounty Kist	89
California	30
La Choy	23
Mixed Vegetables, frozen, Chinese style	
Birds Eye Cantonese	123
Birds Eye International	48
Green Giant	130
La Choy	72
Mixed Vegetables, frozen, European styles	
Birds Eye	
Danish	74

Italian	98
Parisian	74

Mixed Vegetables, frozen, Hawaiian style

Birds Eye	98
Green Giant	197

Mixed Vegetables, frozen, Japanese style

Birds Eye	98
Birds Eye with seasonings	74
Green Giant	130
La Choy, 1 pkg	71

Mixed Vegetables, frozen, American styles

Birds Eye

New England	150
New Orleans Creole	150
Jubilee	250
Pennsylvania Dutch	98
San Francisco	111
Wisconsin	111
Green Giant	130

Mushrooms

Birds Eye	50
Brandywine	30
B & B	60
Dole	5
Green Giant	15

Mustard greens

Birds Eye	44
Seabrook Farms	42

Okra

Birds Eye	61

Green Giant	211
Seabrook Farms	52
Onions	
Birds Eye	64
in cream sauce	239
whole	98
Green Giant	140
Lord Mott	60
in cream sauce	130
Ore-Ida	80
Seabrook Farms	232
Onion Rings, 1 oz	
Birds Eye	170
Mrs. Paul's	60
O & C	178
Ore-Ida	80
Peas, canned	
early	
Del Monte	110
Kounty Kist	139
Le Sueur	110
Lindy	138
Lord Mott	110
Minnesota Valley	109
Stokely-Van Camp	128
sweet	
Del Monte	101
Green Giant	110
with onion	105
Kounty Kist	131

Libby's	121
Lindy	130
S & W	70
Stokely-Van Camp	130
with carrots	
Del Monte	100
Libby's	101
Lord Mott	165
S & W	65
Stokely-Van Camp	120
Peas, frozen	
early	
Birds Eye	169
Green Giant	102
Kounty Kist	119
Le Sueur	149
Seabrook Farms	148
sweet	
Birds Eye	155
Green Giant	150
Seabrook Farms	104
with carrots	
Birds Eye	122
Kounty Kist	90
Seabrook Farms	82
with cream sauce	
Birds Eye	369
Green Giant	300
with cream sauce and cauliflower	
Birds Eye	247

in onion sauce
   Seabrook Farms   192
with onions
   Birds Eye   149
with onions and carrots
   Le Sueur   180
with potatos
   Birds Eye   431
with mushrooms
   Birds Eye   155

Peppers, green
  Stouffers, 1 pkg   225
  Weight Watchers, one 13-oz pkg   320

Potatoes, canned
  Del Monte   90
  Hormel au gratin, 7½-oz can   270
    with ham, 7½-oz can   255
  Stokely-Van Camp   103

Potatoes, frozen, 3 oz unless noted
  Au gratin
    Green Giant, 1 cup   390
    Stouffer's   270
  French fried
    Birds Eye
      Crinkle Cuts   124
      Cottage Fries   120
      Gold Crinkle Cuts   140
      French   111
      Shoestrings   138
      Steak Fries   109

Ore-Ida

Cottage Fries	140
Golden Crinkles	130
Sizzling Fries	157
Sizzling Crinkles	171
Sizzling Shoestrings	218
Shoestrings	170

Hash browns

Birds Eye	54
O'Brien	45
Ore-Ida	70
in butter sauce	120
in butter sauce and onions	130

with parsley

Seabrook Farms	208

Scalloped

Stouffer's	252

Shredded hash browns

Birds Eye	60
Ore-Ida	60

Slices

Green Giant	210

with sour cream

Green Giant	270

Stuffed

Green Giant

with cheese, 5 oz	240
with sour cream, 5 oz	229

with peas

Green Giant	242

Taters and Puffs
  Birds Eye Tasti Fries   140
    Tasti Puffs   190
  Ore-Ida Tater Tots   160
    Tater Tots with Bacon   151
    Tater Tots with Onion   165
With Vermicelli
  Green Giant   399
Whole
  Birds Eye   179
  Ore-Ida   70
  Seabrook Farms   153
Potatoes, mix, ½ cup
  French's   120
    Big Tate   129
    Hungry Jack   160
Julienne
  Betty Crocker   132
Au gratin
  Betty Crocker   150
  French's   190
Creamed
  Betty Crocker   163
Hash browns
  Betty Crocker   147
  French's   160
Pancakes
  French's 3 cakes   130
Potato Buds
  Betty Crocker   132

Scalloped
 Betty Crocker   150
 French's   189
With sour cream
 Betty Crocker   144

Pumpkin
 Del Monte   79
 Libby's   80
 Stokely-Van Camp   88

Sauerkraut
 Del Monte   50
 Libby's   42
 Stokely-Van Camp   50
  Bavarian   69

Soup Greens
 Durkee   213

Spinach, canned
 Del Monte   45
 Libby's   44
 Lord Mott   44

Spinach, frozen
 chopped
  Birds Eye   47
  Seabrook Farms   50
 creamed
  Birds Eye   157
  Green Giant   190
  Lord Mott   130

Seabrook Farms	200
leaf	
Birds Eye	47
Seabrook Farms	48
souffle	
Green Giant	300
Stouffer's, 1 pkg	400
with butter sauce	
Green Giant	89
Squash	
Birds Eye	100
Green Giant	118
Seabrook Farms	92
Stew, vegetable	
Dinty Moore, 7½-oz can	160
Ore-Ida	140
Succotash	
Birds Eye	202
Libby's creamed	190
kernel	151
Seabrook Farms	174
Stokely-Van Camp	170
Sweet Potatoes	
Birds Eye	408
Green Giant	341
Lord Mott	235
Mrs. Paul's	320
Tomatoes	
stewed	70
whole	50

8

Tomato paste
   Contadina   200
   Del Monte   200
   Hunt's   185
   Town House   225
Tomato puree
   Contadina   120
Turnip Greens
   Birds Eye   47
   Seabrook Farms   44
   Stokely-Van Camp   46
Zucchini
   Birds Eye   39
   Del Monte   60
   Mrs. Paul's   480

CHAPTER 9

Condiments, Dips, Dressings, Oils and Sauces

CONDIMENTS,
1 Tbsp, unless noted

celery flakes, 1 tsp
Wyler's   7
curry powder
Crosse & Blackwell   26
garlic flavoring, 1 tsp
Burton's   42
garlic powder, 1 tsp
Wyler's   8
garlic spread
Lawry's   88
horseradish
Borden   16
Heinz   26
Kraft   4
Tastee   5
hot sauce, 1 tsp
Frank's   10
Gebhardt   4
Tabasco   4
meat sauces
A-1   12
Crosse & Blackwell   21
Durkee   60
Escoffier   19
Gravymaster, 1 tsp   8
Heinz 57   14
Heinz Savory   21
H.P.   21
Maggi   17

Steak Supreme	20
mustard	
Brown	
French's	15
Gulden's	13
Heinz	11
Mr. Mustard	11
Dijon	
Grey Poupon	15
German	
Kraft	15
Horseradish	
French's	15
Hot	
Gulden's Diablo	13
Heinz	11
Onion	
French's	25
Yellow	
French's	16
Gulden's	11
Heinz	10
Kraft	12
onion flakes, 1 tsp	
Wyler's	7
onion flavoring, 1 tsp	
Burton's	42
onion powder, 1 tsp	
Wyler's	1

onions, minced, 1 tsp
  Borden's   7
  Wyler's   7
parsley flakes, 1 tsp
  Wyler's   1
pepper
  Seasoned
    Lawry's, 1 tsp   16
  sweet
    Wyler's, 1 tsp   2
salt, flavored, 1 tsp
  celery   6
  garlic   6
  onion   6
sandwich spread
  Hellman's   60
  Kraft   56
vinegar
  Cider or white   1
  Wine
    Holland House
      Marsala   35
      Red   25
      Sherry   40
      White   25
    Regina
      Sauterne   1
      Sherry   10

Flavorings, Extracts, 1 tsp

Almond
Durkee	13
Ehlers	5

Anise
Durkee	16
Ehlers	12

Banana
Durkee	15
Ehlers	7

Black Walnut
Durkee	45

Brandy
Durkee	15
Ehlers	18

Cherry
Ehlers	8

Chocolate
Durkee	8

Coconut
Durkee	7
Ehlers	13

Lemon
Durkee	17
Ehlers	14

Maple
Durkee	6
Ehlers	9

9

Mocha
Durkee 14
Orange
Durkee 16
Ehlers 14
Peppermint
Durkee 15
Ehlers 12
Pineapple
Ehlers 13
Raspberry
Ehlers 10
Rum
Durkee 14
Ehlers 12
Strawberry
Durkee 12
Ehlers 11
Vanilla
Durkee 5

Relishes, Pickles, Olives: 1 piece unless noted

Capers, 1 Tbsp
Crosse & Blackwell 6

Carrots, dill
 Cresca Cocktail Sticks   1
Cauliflower, sweet
 Heinz   9
 Smucker's   23
ChowChow, 1 Tbsp
 Crosse & Blackwell   20
Chutney
 Major Grey's   53
Eggplant
 Cresca   1
Olives
 Green, Manzanilla
  Durkee   4
  Grandee   4
 Green, Spanish
  Vita   11
 Green, queen
  Durkee   14
  Grandee   14
 Ripe
  Durkee   7
  Grandee   7
  Lindsay   6
  Vita   7
Onions
 Cresca   1
 Crosse & Blackwell   1
 Heinz   2
 Heinz Spiced   1

Peppers, 1 oz unless noted
Chili
Del Monte 5
Ortega
Jalapeños 8
Green 5
Hot, 1 pepper
Cresca 6
Smucker's 10
Mild, sweet
Del Monte 5
Pickled
Old El Paso 9
Red, bell
Ortega 9

Pickle Relish, 1 Tbsp
Barbecue
Crosse & Blackwell 22
Heinz 31
Corn
Crosse & Blackwell 15
Hamburger
Crosse & Blackwell 20
Heinz 17
Hot dog
Crosse & Blackwell 22
Heinz 2
Hot pepper
Crosse & Blackwell 22

India
   Crosse & Blackwell   26
piccalilli
   Crosse & Blackwell   25
   Heinz   19

Pickles
  Sour
   Bond's   2
   Crosse & Blackwell   2
   Heinz
     Genuine Dill   10
     Kosher Dills   2
   L & S   2
  Sweet
   Bond's   19
   Crosse & Blackwell   28
     slices, 1 Tbsp   15
   Heinz
     Midget   5
     Sweet Gherkins   25
     Sweet Pickles   45
     Sticks   13
     Candied dill strips   35

Pimientos, 1 oz
  Dromedary   8
  Ortega   7
  Stokely-Van Camp   8

Watermelon Rind, 1 Tbsp   38

9

Seasonings, 1 tsp unless noted

Accent	9
Bacon	
Ann Page	8
Baco's	13
Durkee	3
French's	2
Lawry's	13
McCormick	
Bits	10
Chips	12
Schilling	
Bits	19
Chips	13
Barbecue	
French's	6
Chili Powder	
Lawry's	9
Mexene	8
Cinnamon Sugar	
French's	16
Chutney	
Major Grey's	16
Spice Island	12
Herb	
Lawry's	9
Horseradish	
Reese	18

Hot Sauce
  Frank's 1
Lemon Pepper
  Lawry's 7
  French's 6
Meat Tenderizer
  French's 2
Pepper
  French's 8
  Lawry's 8
Salad
  Durkee 4
    with cheese 10
  French's 6
Salt
  French's
    Butter 8
    Celery 2
    Garlic 4
    Hickory Smoked 2
    Onion 6
    Parsley Garlic 6
    Seasoned 2
  Lawry's
    Garlic 5
    Onion 4
    Seasoned 1
Seafood
  French's 2

227

Stock Base
    French's   8

Seasoning Mixes, 1 pkg, various sizes

A la King
    Durkee   297
Beef
    Lawry's
        Beef Olé   126
        Marinade   69
Beef Stew
    Durkee   99
    French's   150
    Lawry's   131
    McCormick   90
    Schilling   89
Beef Stroganoff
    French's   192
    Lawry's   119
    McCormick   113
Beef, Ground
    Ann Page   100
    Durkee   91
    French's   100
Chili
    Ann Page   120
    French's   150

Pizza 99
French's 128
Lawry's 139
McCormick 167
Schilling 172
Rice, Fried
Durkee 62
Rice, Spanish
Durkee 129
Lawry's 125
Swiss Steak
McCormick 44
Schilling 42
Taco
Durkee 67
French's 150
McCormick 65
Schilling 65
Tuna Casserole
McCormick 104

DIPS, 1 oz

Ready to Serve

Bacon and Horseradish
Borden   79
Kraft
  Ready   71
  Teez   57
Lucerne   63
Bacon and Smoke
Sealtest   47
Barbecue
Borden's   48
Bean
Chili
  Lucerne   50
Jalapeño
  Frito-Lay   36
  Gebhardt   30
  Granny Goose   37
  Lucerne   35
Blue Cheese
Granny Goose   110
Kraft
  Ready   69
  Teez   51

Lucerne 67
Sealtest 49

Casino
Sealtest 45

Chili, Green
Borden 55

Chipped Beef
Sealtest 44

Clam
Kraft
Ready 66
Teez 44
Lucerne 34

Clam and Lobster
Borden 60

Dill
Kraft 67

Garlic
Granny Goose 100
Kraft 47
Lucerne 58

Green Goddess
Kraft 45

Guacamole
Lucerne 69

Hickory Smoke
Lucerne 60

Onion
Borden 48
Lawry's 50

   Kraft
      Ready   68
      Teez   43
   Lucerne   58
   Sealtest   46
Tartar
   Borden   48

Unprepared Mixes

Bacon and Onion
   Frito-Lay   100
Barbecue
   Salada   120
Blue Cheese
   Frito-Lay   117
   Lawry's   94
Caesar
   Frito-Lay   118
   Lawry's   94
Cheddar Cheese
   Salada   43
Chili
   Frito-Lay   120
Dill
   Frito-Lay   90
Dill and Chives
   Salada   130

Garlic and Onion

McCormick	126
Salada	100

Horseradish

Lawry's	86
Frito-Lay	105

Onion

Frito-Lay	87
Green	100
Lawry's	
Green	100
Toasted	82
McCormick	131
Salada	100

Taco

Frito-Lay	105

SALAD DRESSINGS,
1 Tbsp unless noted

Avocado

Kraft	70

Bacon

Lawry's	78

Blue Cheese

Ann Page Low Calorie	18

Kraft
  Chunky   70
  Low Calorie   14
  Low Calorie Chunky   30
Lawry's
  bottled   57
  mix, 1 pkg   74
Nu Made   75
Roka   60
Seven Seas   70
Wish-Bone   80
Weight Watchers   10

Caesar
Kraft   70
Lawry's
  bottled   70
  mix, 1 pkg   72
Nu Made   75
Pfeiffer   70
  Low Calorie   10
Seven Seas   70
Wish-Bone   80

Chef Style
Ann Page   20
Kraft   18

Coach House
Seven Seas   78

Coleslaw
Kraft   70
  Low Calorie   30

Cucumber
  Kraft   80
    Low Calorie   30
French
  Ann Page   25
  Casino   70
  Kraft   60
    Casino Garlic   70
    Herb and Garlic   90
    Low Calorie   25
    Miracle   70
  Lawry's
    bottled   50
    mix, 1 pkg   72
  Nu Made
    Low Calorie   20
    Savory   65
    Zesty   70
  Pfeiffer   55
    Low Calorie   18
  Seven Seas   60
    Low Calorie   30
  Tillie Lewis   12
  Wish-Bone
    Deluxe   50
    French Garlic   70
    Low Calorie   25
    Sweet and Spicy   70
  Weight Watchers   4

Garlic
Kraft	50
Wish-Bone	80

Green Goddess
Kraft	80
Lawry's	
bottled	60
mix, 1 pkg	69
Nu Made	80
Seven Seas	80
Wish-Bone	60

Green Onion
Kraft	70

Hawaiian
Lawry's	75

Herb and Garlic
Kraft	83

Herb and Spices
Seven Seas	60

Italian
Ann Page	14
Good Seasons	8
Kraft	80
Golden	70
Low Calorie	6
Lawry's	
bottled	80
mix, 1 pkg	44
cheeses mix, 1 pkg	69

Nu Made	90
Low Calorie	16
Pfeiffer	60
Low Calorie	10
Seven Seas	70
Family	60
Low Calorie	35
Viva	70
Tillie Lewis	6
Weight Watchers	2
Wish-Bone	80
Low Calorie	20
Lemon garlic	
Lawry's, 1 pkg	65
Mayonnaise, all brands	100
Mayonnaise, flavored	
Durkee	69
Mayonnaise, imitation	
Mrs. Filbert's	40
Piedmont	50
Weight Watchers	40
May Lo Naise	
Tillie Lewis	25
Oil and Vinegar	
Kraft	70
Lawry's	55
Nu Made	60
Seven Seasons	70
Onion	
Lawry's	84

Wish-Bone	80
Parmesan	
Good Seasons	84
Roquefort	
Kraft	58
Red Wine	
Pfeiffer	40
Low Calorie	10
Russian	
Kraft	30
Nu Made	55
Pfeiffer	65
Low Calorie	15
Seven Seas	80
Tillie Lewis	12
Weight Watchers	
bottled	50
mix	4
Wish-Bone	60
Low Calorie	25
Salad dressing	
Ann Page	70
Heinz	63
Kraft	65
Mrs. Filbert's	65
Nu Made	80
Piedmont	70
Sultana	50
Salad Secret	
Kraft	60

9

Sea Island
Kraft   93
Sour Treat
Friendship   90
Sherry
Lawry's   55
Spin Blend
Hellmann's   55
Tahitian Isle
Wish-Bone   55
Thousand Island
Ann Page   25
Kraft   60
  Low Calorie   30
Lawry's
  bottled   65
  mix, 1 pkg   78
Nu Made   30
Pfeiffer   65
  Low Calorie   15
Seven Seas   50
Tillie Lewis   18
Weight Watchers
  bottled   50
  mix   12
Wish-Bone   70
  Low Calorie   25
Tomato-Blue Cheese
Kraft   90

Tomato-Spice
Seven Seas 45
Whipped
Tillie Lewis 25
Yogonaise
Henri's 60
Yogowhip
Henri's 60
Yogurt, all flavors
Henri's 35

OILS, 1 Tbsp

Corn
Mazola 122
Nu Made 124
Olive
Filippo Berio 125
Peanut
Planters 128
Popcorn
Planters 130
Safflower
Nu Made 119
Soybean
Mrs. Tucker's 128

Sunflower
Sunlight   120
Vegetable
Crisco   120
Puritan   118
Swift   115
Wesson   120
Vegetable and cottonseed
Swift   120

Shortening, 1 Tbsp unless noted

Lard   115
1 cup   1,850
Vegetable
Crisco   109
Fluffo   109
Mrs. Tucker's   120
Pam   7
Snowdrift   111
Spry   97

SAUCES,
½ cup unless noted

A la King
  Durkee — 66
Barbecue, 1 Tbsp
  Chris' and Pitt's — 15
  Durkee with vinegar — 64
  French's — 14
    Hot — 27
    Smoky — 14
  Open Pit — 26
    Hot 'n Spicy — 27
    Hickory Smoked — 27
    with onions — 28
Bearnaise
  Butternut Farm — 176
Bordelaise
  Butternut Farm — 48
Cheese
  Durkee — 168
  French's — 160
  McCormick — 156
  Schilling — 156
Chili
  Gebhardt — 156
  Heinz — 17

9

Hunt's	18
McCormick	92
Clam	
Buitoni	
red	102
white	114
La Rosa	
red	78
white	68
Cocktail Sauce	
Crosse & Blackwell	26
Tastee	25
Enchilada	
Gebhardt	68
Lawry's, 1 pkg	144
McCormick, 1 pkg	116
Old El Paso	
Hot	36
Mild	40
Hollandaise	
Durkee	118
French's	119
McCormick	171
Schilling	170
Horseradish, 1 oz	
Kraft	100
Italian	
Contadina	85
Lawry's, 1 pkg	86
Ragu	36

Lemon-Butter, 1 oz
  Weight Watchers   16
Mint Sauce, 1 tsp
  Crosse & Blackwell   16
Mushroom, 1 oz
  Dawn Fresh   9
Pizza
  Buitoni   92
  Ragu   96
Seafood cocktail sauce, 1 tsp
  Del Monte   18
  Pfeiffer   25
Sour Cream
  Durkee   160
  French's   280
  McCormick   146
  Schilling   146
Soy Sauce, 1 tsp
  La Choy   7
Spaghetti
  Ann Page   70
    Marinara   70
    Meat   80
    Mix, 1 envelope   120
    with Mushrooms   70
  Buitoni   92
    Clam, red   108
    Clam, white   144
    Marinara   88
    Meat   120

with Mushrooms	88
Durkee	45
with Mushrooms	40
French's	80
with Mushrooms	80
Franco-American	95
with Mushrooms	95
Lawry's	147
with Meatball seasoning	316
with Mushrooms	116
La Rosa	74
Prince	90
with Meat	143
with Mushrooms	103
Ragu	
Plain	96
Thick	84
Clam	88
Marinara	96
Meat	92
Thick with Meatball seasoning	104
with Mushrooms	84
Spatini	51
Town House	80
with Meat	80
with Mushrooms	89
Stroganoff	
Durkee	410
French's	165
Lawry's, 1 pkg	118

McCormick	115
Schilling	115
Sweet and Sour	
Contadina	158
Durkee	115
French's	55
La Choy	262
Swiss Steak	
Contadina	48
Taco Sauce	
Gebhardt	3
Old El Paso	4
Tartar Sauce	
Best Foods	70
Hellman's	75
Kraft	72
Lawry's	67
Seven Seas	80
Teriyaki, 1 Tbsp	
Chun King	12
French's	17
Tomato	
Contadina	45
Del Monte	40
with Bits	40
with Mushrooms	50
with Onions	50
Hunt's	35
Prima Salsa	109
Prima Salsa with Mushrooms	110

Special	40
with Bits	35
with Cheese	71
with Herbs	80
with Meat	120
with Mushrooms	40
with Onions	45
Stokely-Van Camp	35
Town House	40
Tomato Paste	
Contadina	46
Hunt's	108
Lord Mott	44
Tuna Casserole	
McCormick	128
Schilling	128
White	
Durkee	119
Wine, 1 oz	
Lawry's	
Burgundy	98
Sherry	94
White	113
Worcestershire Sauce	
Crosse & Blackwell	15
Heinz	11
French's	10
Lea & Perrins	12

Gravies, ¼ cup unless noted

Au Jus
Ann Page 1 envelope	64
Durkee	8
Durkee, Roastin' Bag, 1 pkg	64
French's	8
French's Pan Rich	30
McCormick	4
Schilling	4

Beef
Franco-American	30
Howard Johnson's	25
Wyler's	24

Brown
Ann Page 1 envelope	79
Dawn Fresh	20
Durkee	15
with Mushrooms	15
with Onions	17
Franco-American	25
French's	20
French's Pan Rich	62
McCormick	26
Herb	21
Lite	10
Pillsbury	15
Schilling	26
Herb	21

Weight Watchers   8
  with Mushrooms   12
  with Onions   13
Chicken
 Ann Page, 1 envelope   120
 College Inn   25
 Durkee   22
  Creamy   39
  Roastin' Bag, 1 pkg   122
  Roastin' Bag Italian, 1 pkg   144
 French's   25
 French's Pan Rich   60
 McCormick   21
  Lite   10
 Pillsbury   25
 Schilling   21
  Lite   10
 Weight Watchers   10
 Wyler's   24
Chicken Giblet
 Franco-American   35
Herb
 McCormick   26
Homestyle
 Durkee   18
 French's   25
 Pillsbury   15
Meatloaf
 Durkee, 1 pkg   130

Mushroom
Ann Page, 1 envelope	79
Durkee	16
Franco-American	35
French's	20
McCormick	19
Schilling	19
Wyler's	15

Mustard
French's	16

Onion
Ann Page, 1 envelope	120
Durkee	21
Durkee Roastin' Bag, 1 pkg	124
French's	25
French's Pan Rich	50

Pork
Durkee	18
Durkee Roastin' Bag, 1 pkg	130
French's	20

Pot Roast
Durkee, 1 pkg	124

Sparerib
Durkee, 1 pkg	162

Swiss Steak
Durkee	11
Durkee Roastin' Bag, 1 pkg	115

Turkey
Durkee	23

CHAPTER 10

Desserts, Baking and Baked Goods

BAKING MISCELLANY

10

Baking Chocolate, 1 oz
  Chips
    Baker's   130
    Hershey's   115
    Nestlé   130
  Ground
    Ghiradelli   150
  Solid
    Baker's
      German   140
      semi-sweet   130
      unsweetened   140
    Ghiradelli   150
    Hershey   190
Butterscotch
  Nestlé chips   150
Coconut
  Baker's   150
Ginger
  Borden's crystallized   98
  Borden's preserved   88
Peanut Butter
  Reese chips   150

CAKES, FROZEN,
1 whole cake

Banana
Pepperidge Farm 1,115
Sara Lee 1,439
Banana Nut
Sara Lee 1,864
Black Forest
Sara Lee 1,625
Boston Creme
Pepperidge Farm 1,070
Cheesecake
Lambrecht 1,530
Mrs. Smith's 1,230
Sara Lee
small 860
large 1,440
Cherry 1,280
French 2,190
Strawberry 1,280
Strawberry French 2,062
Chocolate
Pepperidge Farm 1,238
Sara Lee 1,380
Chocolate Bavarian
Sara Lee 2,250

Chocolate Fudge
Pepperidge Farm — 1,800
Chocolate, German
Pepperidge Farm — 1,589
Sara Lee — 1,234
Coconut
Pepperidge Farm — 1,800
Crumbcake
Sara Lee — 170
Stouffer's
   Blueberry — 211
   Chocolate Chip — 225
   French — 200
Cupcake
Stouffer's
   Cream — 240
   Yellow — 190
Devil's Food
Pepperidge Farm — 1,800
Sara Lee — 1,496
Golden
Pepperidge Farm — 900
Sara Lee — 1,440
Lemon
Sara Lee — 2,175
Lemon Coconut
Pepperidge Farm — 1,100
Mandarin Orange
Sara Lee — 1,650

Orange
  Howard Johnson's — 1,700
  Sara Lee — 1,440
Pound
  Sara Lee
    Banana Nut — 1,170
    Chocolate — 1,220
    Chocolate Swirl — 1,300
    Plain — 1,320
    Raisin — 1,270
  Pepperidge Farm
    Apple Nut — 1,300
    Butter — 1,300
    Carrot — 1,600
    Chocolate — 1,300
Cherry
  Mrs. Smith's — 2,335
Strawberry
  Mrs. Smith's — 1,830
  Sara Lee — 1,550
    Strawberry and Cream — 1,700
Vanilla
  Pepperidge Farm — 1,900
Walnut
  Sara Lee — 1,690

CAKE MIXES, 1 whole cake

Angel Food
Betty Crocker	1,560
One Step	1,680
Confetti	1,800
Strawberry	1,800
Duncan Hines	1,670
Pillsbury	1,680
Swans Down	1,590

Apple Raisin
Duncan Hines	2,280
Spicy	1,620

Applesauce Raisin
Betty Crocker	1,800

Banana
Betty Crocker	3,140
Duncan Hines	2,400
Pillsbury	3,120

Banana Nut
Betty Crocker	1,800
Duncan Hines	1,800

Bundt
Pillsbury	
Fudge	3,480
Lemon	3,350
Macaroon	3,950
Marble	3,960

Pound	3,710
Triple Fudge	3,590

Butter

Duncan Hines	3,240
Pillsbury	2,680

Butter Brickle

Betty Crocker	3,110

Butter Fudge

Duncan Hines	3,240

Butter Pecan

Betty Crocker	3,120

Cheesecake

Jello-O	2,000
Pillsbury	3,120
Royal	1,840

Cherry

Duncan Hines	2,280

Cherry Chip

Betty Crocker	2,280

Chocolate

Betty Crocker	1,380
Duncan Hines	2,400
Pillsbury Dark	3,120
Swans Down	2,240

Chocolate Almond

Betty Crocker	1,890

Chocolate Chip

Betty Crocker	1,980
Duncan Hines	1,710
Double Chocolate Chip	1,620

Chocolate Fudge
  Betty Crocker   3,240
Chocolate, German
  Betty Crocker   3,240
  Pillsbury   3,120
Chocolate, Sour Cream
  Betty Crocker   3,240
  Duncan Hines   2,400
Chocolate, Swiss
  Duncan Hines   2,400
  Swans Down   2,240
Chocolate with frosting
  Betty Crocker   1,620
Coconut Pecan
  Betty Crocker   1,975
Date Nut
  Betty Crocker   1,890
Devil's Food
  Betty Crocker   3,240
  Duncan Hines   2,400
  Pillsbury   3,240
  Swans Down   2,230
Fudge Marble
  Duncan Hines   2,400
  Pillsbury   3,240
Gingerbread
  Betty Crocker   1,890
Lemon
  Betty Crocker   3,240
    Pudding Cake   1,380

Duncan Hines	2,400
Pillsbury	3,240

Lemon Chiffon

Betty Crocker	2,280

Marble

Betty Crocker	3,280

Orange

Betty Crocker	3,240
Duncan Hines	2,400

Pineapple

Betty Crocker	2,400
Duncan Hines	2,400

Pound

Betty Crocker	2,280

Spice

Betty Crocker	3,240
Duncan Hines	2,400

Spice Raisin

Betty Crocker	1,800

Strawberry

Betty Crocker	3,240
Duncan Hines	2,400

Streusel

Pillsbury

Cinnamon	4,080
Devil's Food	3,950
Fudge Marble	4,080
Chocolate	3,950
Lemon	4,200

10

White

Betty Crocker	2,400
Duncan Hines	2,280
Pillsbury	3,000
Swans Down	2,120

Yellow

Betty Crocker	3,240
Butter	2,880
with frosting	1,380
Duncan Hines	2,400
Pillsbury	3,120
Swans Down	2,240

CAKES FOR SNACKS, 1 cake

Big Wheels	170
Brownie	
Hostess	
small	150
large	240
Chocolate, cream-filled	
Yankee Doodles	134
Choco-Diles	250
Creamies, 1 pkg	
Tastykake	
Chocolate	255

Spice	270
Crumb Cakes	
Hostess	130
Cupcakes	
Hostess	
Chocolate	155
Orange	147
Tastykake, 1 pkg	
Buttercream	238
Chocolate	200
Chocolate Cream	239
Devil Dogs	169
Devil's Food	
Hostess	140
Drake's	135
Ding Dongs	170
Donuts	
Hostess	
Cinnamon	110
Crunch	100
Enrobed	130
Plain	105
Powdered	115
Funny Bones, 1 pkg	162
Ho-Ho's	120
Juniors, 1 pkg	
Tastykake	
Chocolate	307
Coconut	330
Coffee cake	310

10

Krimpets, 1 pkg
  Tastykake
    Butterscotch   190
    Chocolate   255
    Jelly   168
    Vanilla   240
Macaroons
  Hostess   210
Oatmeal Raisin, 1 pkg
  Tastykake   267
Orange Treats, 1 pkg
  Tastykake   230
Pound
  Drake's
    Marble   185
    Plain   181
    Raisin   323
Ring Ding   366
Sno Balls   140
Tandy Takes, 1 pkg
  Chocolate   180
  Peanut Butter   190
Teens, 1 pkg   225
Tempty, 1 pkg
  Chocolate   196
  Lemon   259
Tiger Tails   415
Twinkies   140

COFFEE CAKE, 1 cake

Almond
Sara Lee	1,350
Sara Lee Coffee Ring	1,100

Angel Food
Howard Johnson's	710

Apple
Morton	1,130
Sara Lee	1,175

Apple Cinnamon
Pillsbury	1,880

Apricot
Sara Lee	1,176

Banana
Sara Lee	1,440

Blueberry
Sara Lee Coffee Ring	1,080
Sara Lee Danish	1,175

Butter Pecan
Pillsbury	2,480

Butter Streusel
Sara Lee	1,395

Cherry
Sara Lee	1,050

Chocolate
Sara Lee	1,375

10

Chocolate, German
Morton	1,360
Sara Lee	1,230

Cinnamon Streusel
Pillsbury	2,000
Sara Lee	1,230

Coconut
Pepperidge Farm	1,940

Coffee Cake
Aunt Jemima	1,360

Crumb
Drake's	1,460

Lemon
Drake's	1,030

Maple Crunch
Sara Lee	1,157

Orange
Sara Lee	1,442

Pecan
Drake's	1,109
Morton	1,368
Sara Lee small	764
Sara Lee large	1,320

Raspberry
Sara Lee	1,090

Sour Cream
Pillsbury	2,160

COOKIES, 1 piece

Adelaide
Pepperidge Farm	53

Almond
Keebler	47
Stella D'Oro	49

Almond Spice
Keebler	50

Angel Puffs
Stella D'Oro	17

Animal Crackers
Keebler	12
Nabisco	12
Sunshine	10

Animal Crackers Iced
Keebler	52
Sunshine	26

Anise
Stella D'Oro
Anisette Sponge	50
Anisette Toast	34

Apple
Keebler	27
Nabisco	48

Applesauce
Sunshine
	33
Iced	104

Arrowroot
 Nabisco   22
 Sunshine   16
Assorted
 Stella D'Oro
  Hostess   39
  Lady Stella   37
Bordeaux
 Pepperidge Farm   37
Breakfast Treats
 Stella D'Oro   100
Brown Edge
 Nabisco   28
Brown Sugar
 Nabisco   25
 Pepperidge Farm   50
Brussels
 Pepperidge Farm   57
Butter
 Keebler   84
 Nabisco   37
 Pepperidge Farm   38
 Sunshine   24
Capri
 Pepperidge Farm   85
Cashew
 Nabisco   57
Chessman
 Pepperidge Farm   43

Chinese Dessert
  Stella D'Oro 170
Chocolate
  Keebler
    Bavarian Fudge 80
    Nut Fudge 31
    Pecan Fudge 66
  Melody 31
  Nabisco
    Wafers 28
    Snaps 18
  Pepperidge Farm 48
  Sunshine 13
Chocolate Almond
  Nabisco 55
Chocolate Brownies
  Pepperidge Farm 57
Chocolate Chip
  Chips Ahoy 50
  Estee 30
  Keebler 44
    Old Fashioned 80
    Rich 'N Chips 73
    Townhouse 49
  Nabisco 51
    Family Favorite 33
    Snaps 21
  Pepperidge Farm 52
  Sunshine 37
  Chip-A-Roos 63

Chocolate Chip Coconut
Keebler	80
Nabisco	76
Sunshine	76

Chocolate Strawberry Wafers
Estee	90

Cinnamon
Sunshine	20

Cinnamon Almond
Nabisco	53

Cinnamon Sugar
Fun Days	48
Pepperidge Farm	52

Coconut
Keebler	61
Old Fashioned	83
Strip	37
Nabisco	16
Stella D'Oro	47
Sunshine	47

Coconut, Iced
Keebler Crunchies	70

Coconut Chocolate
Pepperidge Farm	83

Creme Sandwiches
Butterscotch	
Keebler	85
Chocolate	
Keebler Dutch	95

Keebler Opera	85
Oreo grocery	50
Oreo individual	40
Chocolate fudge	
Cookie Mates	53
Keebler	97
Sunshine	74
Coconut	
Nabisco	53
Sunshine	51
Wise Coco	39
Lemon	
Keebler	85
Swiss	
Nabisco	43
Vanilla	
Cameo	68
Cookie Mates	52
Keebler	82
French	95
Opera	85
Sunshine	79
Vienna Fingers	69
Wise	38
Crescents	
Nabisco	34
Cup Custard	
Sunshine	70
Danish Wedding	
Keebler	31

Date Nut
Pepperidge Farm	53
Sunshine	82

Devil's Food
Keebler	64
Nabisco	58
Sunshine	55

Dixie Vanilla
Sunshine	60

Egg Biscuits
Stella D'Oro	37
Anise	135
Egg Jumbo	43
Rum and Brandy	135
Sugared	135
Vanilla	130

Figs
Nabisco Fig Newtons	59
Frito-Lay	189
Keebler	71
Sunshine	42

Fruit
Stella D'Oro	67
Sunshine Golden Fruit	61

Fruit, Iced
Nabisco	70

Fudge
Keebler	
Sticks	42

Strips	57
Pepperidge Farm	58
Gingerbread	
Pepperidge Farm	33
Gingerbread, Iced	
Keebler	130
Ginger Snaps	
Keebler	39
Nabisco	30
Sunshine	
small	14
large	32
Golden Bars	
Stella D'Oro	110
Graham Crackers	
Keebler	
Honey	17
Thin	17
Very Thin	14
Nabisco	30
Honey Maid	30
Sunshine	17
Sugar Honey	30
Graham Crackers, chocolate covered	
Keebler	44
Milco	91
Nabisco	55
Fancy Dip	68
Pantry	62
Robena	72

Kichel
   Stella D'Oro   64
Lady Joan
   Sunshine   42
   Sunshine Iced   47
LaLanne
   Sunshine   15
Lemon
   Keebler   83
   Nabisco   17
   Sunshine   76
      Lemon Coolers   29
Lemon Nut
   Pepperidge Farm   58
Lido
   Pepperidge Farm   95
Love Cookies
   Stella D'Oro   110
Macaroons
   Sunshine   85
      Butter   39
      Coconut   81
   Bake Shop   87
   Nabisco   71
Mandel Toast
   Stella D'Oro   54
Margherite
   Stella D'Oro   73
Marigold Sandwich
   Keebler   91

Marshmallow
Chocolate covered
Keebler
Dainties 68
Galaxies 82
Treasures 83
Tulips 83
Coconut
Nabisco 54
Sunshine 70
Iced
Sunshine
Frosted Cakes 68
Nut Sundae 74
Mallomars 60
Nabisco
Puffs 94
Twirls 133
Pinwheels 139
Sunshine
Puffs 63
Kings 135
Sandwich
Keebler 81
Nabisco 32
Sprinkles
Sunshine 71
Milano
Pepperidge Farm 63
Mint 70

Peanut Butter
Keebler	81
Nabisco Nutter Butter	69
Sunshine	
Crunch	68
Patties	30

Peanut Butter, Chocolate-covered
Eton	53
Keebler	117

Peanut Caramel
Hey Days	122

Peanut Cream
Nabisco	34

Pecan
Keebler	20
Sunshine	78

Pfeffernusse
Stella D'Oro	44

Pirouette
Pepperidge Farm	40

Prune
Stella D'Oro	87

Raisin
Nabisco	56
Stella D'Oro	115
Sunshine	73

Raisin, Iced
Keebler	81

Raisin Bran
Pepperidge Farm   53

Shortbread
Keebler   27
Lorna Doone   38
Pepperidge Farm   65
Scottie   39

Shortbread with Cashews
Nabisco   50

Shortbread, Chocolate-covered
Nabisco   50

Shortbread with Coconut   65

Shortbread, Iced   58

Shortbread Pecans
Keebler   77
Nabisco   77

St. Moritz
Pepperidge Farm   47

Sorrento
Stella D'Oro   57

Sprinkles
Sunshine   57

Sugar
Eton   50
Keebler
  Giant   70
  Old Fashioned   81
Nabisco   17
Pepperidge Farm   53

Sugar Wafers
Nabisco Biscos	18
Creme Waffles	47
Keebler	26
Kreemlined	45
Regent	23
Sunshine	47

Sugar Wafers, Chocolate-covered
Eton	54
Milco	80
Nabisco	76
Creme Stix	50
Sunshine	30

Sugar Wafers, Spiced
Nabisco	33

Sunflower Raisin
Pepperidge Farm	53

Swedish Creme	103
Swiss Chalet	97

Swiss Fudge
Stella D'Oro	64

Tahiti
Pepperidge Farm	85

Taste of Vienna
Stella D'Oro	85

Tea Biscuits
Nabisco	21

Toy Cookies
Sunshine	13

Vanilla
  Keebler   19
  Nabisco
    Snaps   13
    Wafers   18
  Sunshine   15
Vanilla Thins
  Estee   25
Vienna Finger Sandwich
  Sunshine   71
Yum Yums
  Sunshine   83
Zanzibar
  Pepperidge Farm   37

PASTRY, FROZEN, MIXES, AND TOASTER, 1 piece unless noted

Dessert mixes
  Pillsbury Appleasy   160
Donuts
  Morton
    Bavarian Creme   180
    Boston Creme   205

Chocolate	150
Glazed	150
Jelly	180
Mini	120
Town House Cinnamon	210
Dumplings, apple	
Pepperidge Farm	280
Strudel, apple	
Pepperidge Farm, 1 oz	85
Tarts	
Kellogg's Pop Tarts	210
Pepperidge Farm	
Apple	280
Blueberry	285
Cherry	280
Lemon	310
Raspberry	320
Popovers (Flako)	166
Turnovers	
Pepperidge Farm	320
Pillsbury	180

PIES, FROZEN, 1 whole pie

Apple	
Banquet	1,440

10

Morton	1,740
Mini	590
Mrs. Smith's	1,768
Natural	2,881
Dutch	1,860
Tart	1,495
Banana Cream	
Banquet	1,032
Morton	1,020
Mini	230
Mrs. Smith's	1,290
Light	1,320
Blueberry	
Banquet	1,523
Morton	1,680
Mini	580
Mrs. Smith's	1,740
Natural	2,040
Boston Cream	
Mrs. Smith's	1,980
Cherry	
Banquet	1,360
Morton	1,805
Mini	591
Mrs. Smith's	1,860
Natural	2,040
Chocolate	
Mrs. Smith's	1,500
Royal Dutch	2,040

Chocolate Cream
Banquet	1,060
Morton	1,200
Mini	260
Mrs. Smith's	1,470

Coconut
Mrs. Smith's	1,380

Coconut Cream
Banquet	1,040
Morton	1,140
Mini	260
Mrs. Smith's	1,380

Coconut Custard
Banquet	1,220
Morton	
Mini	370
Mrs. Smith's	1,590

Custard
Banquet	1,240

Devil Cream
Royal	2,280
Mrs. Smith's	1,470

Lemon
Mrs. Smith's	2,040
Royal	2,080

Lemon Cream
Banquet	1,000
Morton	1,000
Mini	240
Mrs. Smith's	1,350

10

Lemon Crunch
Mrs. Smith's   2,480
Lemon Meringue
Mrs. Smith's   1,560
Lemon Yogurt
Mrs. Smith's   1,200
Mince
Morton   1,860
  Mini   590
Mrs. Smith's   2,010
Mincemeat
Banquet   1,520
Neapolitan Cream
Morton   1,140
Mrs. Smith's   1,440
Nesselrode
Royal   2,000
Peach
Banquet   1,320
Morton   1,680
  Mini   560
Mrs. Smith's   1,800
  Natural   1,980
Pecan
Morton
  Mini   580
Mrs. Smith's   2,589
Pineapple
Mrs. Smith's   1,800

Pineapple-Cheese
   Mrs. Smith's   1,580
Pumpkin
   Banquet   1,230
   Morton   1,380
     Mini   430
   Mrs. Smith's   1,440
Raisin
   Mrs. Smith's   1,890
Spumoni
   Royal   2,120
Strawberry Cream
   Banquet   1,020
   Morton   1,080
   Mrs. Smith's   1,320
Strawberry and Rhubarb
   Mrs. Smith's   1,890
     Natural   1,920
Strawberry-Yogurt
   Mrs. Smith's   1,220

Pie Mixes, 1 whole pie

   Betty Crocker Boston Cream   2,080
   Pillsbury
     Chocolate Cream   2,460
     Lemon Chiffon   1,980
     Vanilla   2,340

10

Pie Crusts and Shells, 1 piece

Pastry Sheets
Pepperidge Farm   570
Pastry Shells
Pepperidge Farm   240
Stella D'Oro   146
Pie Crusts
Betty Crocker   1,920
  Stick   960
Flako   1,560
Pillsbury   1,740
Pie Shells
Pepperidge Farm   521
  shallow   440
  with top   760
Stella D'Oro   240
Tart Shells
Pepperidge Farm   88

Pie Fillings, 1 whole can unless noted

Apple
Wilderness   660
Apricot
Wilderness   720
Banana Cream
Jell-O   660

Blueberry
Wilderness 660
Cherry
Wilderness 650
Lemon
Jell-O 1,080
Royal, 1 cup 310
Wilderness 840
Lime
Royal, 1 cup 310
Mince
Wilderness 840
Mincemeat
None Such, 1 cup 660
Peach
Wilderness 655
Pumpkin
Libby's, 1 cup 205
Stokely-Van Camp, 1 cup 370
Raisin
Wilderness 720
Strawberry
Wilderness 710

10
SMALL PASTRY PIES, 1 piece

Apple
Stella D'Oro	90
Hostess	400
Tastykake	350
Tastykake French	400

Blueberry
Hostess	365

Cherry
Hostess	420
Tastykake	380

Fig
Stella D'Oro	100

Guava
Stella D'Oro	125

Lemon
Hostess	420
Tastykake	355

Peach/Apricot
Stella D'Oro	90

Pecan
Frito-Lay	345

Prune
Stella D'Oro	92

Puff Pastry
Durkee	
Beef	47

Cheese	59
Chicken	49
Chicken liver	48
Shrimp	44

PUDDINGS, MIXES AND CANNED, ½ cup, unless noted

Banana
Ann Page	250
Del Monte	180
Shak-A-Pudd'n	165
Royal	164

Banana Cream
Jell-O	175
My-T-Fine	175

Bavarian Cream
My-T-Fine	176

Butter Pecan
My-T-Fine	175

Butterscotch
Ann Page	190
Instant	170
Del Monte	175

D-Zerta	25
Foremost	175
Jell-O	172
My-T-Fine	170
Royal	190
Sego	250
Caramel Nut	
Royal	195
Cherry	
Whip 'n Chill	139
Cherry-Plum	
Junket	135
Chocolate	
Ann Page	180
Betty Crocker	180
Bounty	174
Dannon	150
Del Monte	250
D-Zerta	20
Foremost	175
Jell-O	175
Instant	190
My-T-Fine	185
Royal	190
Dark 'N Sweet	200
Sego	250
Shak-A-Pudd'n	200
Whip 'n Chill	145
Chocolate Almond	
My-T-Fine	196

Chocolate Fudge

Betty Crocker	180
Del Monte	190
Foremost	175
Jell-O	175
Instant	191
My-T-Fine	190
Sego	250
Whip 'n Chill	139

Chocolate Malt

Shak-A-Pudd'n	200

Chocolate Marshmallow

Sego	250

Coconut

Ann Page	
Cream	190
Toasted	170
Jell-O	175
Instant	190
Royal	185

Currant-Raspberry

Junket	135

Custard

Ann Page	150
Jell-O	165
My-T-Fine	
Caramel	145
Vanilla	156
Rice-A-Roni	120
Royal	145

10

Indian
  B & M 150
Lemon
  Ann Page 150
    Instant 180
  Bounty 196
  Foremost 197
  Jell-O 178
    Instant 179
  My-T-Fine 180
  Royal 180
  Whip 'n Chill 135
Lemon Chiffon
  Jell-O 144
Mocha Nut
  Royal 190
Pineapple Cream
  Jell-O 165
    Instant 179
Pistachio
  Ann Page 180
  Royal 180
Plum
  Crosse & Blackwell 255
  R & R 300
Rice
  Betty Crocker 150
  Bounty 195
Strawberry
  Junket 135

10

Shak-A-Pudd'n	160
Whip 'n Chill	135
Tapioca	
Chocolate	
Ann Page	180
Jell-O	165
Royal	185
Lemon	
Jell-O	166
Orange	
Jell-O	166
Vanilla	
Ann Page	170
Betty Crocker	150
Jell-O	166
My-T-Fine	144
Royal	170
Vanilla	
Ann Page	170
Betty Crocker	190
Bounty	128
Dannon	150
Del Monte	190
D-Zerta	30
Foremost	175
Jell-O	164
Instant	178
My-T-Fine	170
Royal	165
Instant	180

293

Sego	250
Shak-A-Pudd'n	165
Whip 'n Chill	135

CHAPTER 11

Jellies, Syrups, Toppings and Spreads

DESSERT TOPPINGS, 1 Tbsp

Black Cherry
No-Cal   0
Black Raspberry
No-Cal   0
Butterscotch
Hershey's   55
Kraft   60
Smucker's   69
Caramel
Kraft
  chocolate   56

Grape
  No-Cal   0
Hard Sauce
  Crosse & Blackwell   64
Marshmallow
  Kraft   35
Pecans in Syrup
  Kraft   82
  Smucker's   65
Pineapple
  Kraft   50
  Smucker's   62
Strawberry
  Kraft   45
  No-Cal   0
  Smucker's   60
Walnut
  Kraft   88
Walnuts in Syrup
  Smucker's   65
Whip, non-dairy
  Cool Whip   14
  D-Zerta   8
  Dream Whip   10
  Kraft   9
  Lucky Whip   11
  Pet   16
  Reddi-Whip   9

FROSTINGS, 1 can

Betty Crocker
Chocolate Fudge	1920
Coconut Pecan	1310
White, creamy	1920
White, fluffy *Lite*	720
All other flavors	1800

Pillsbury
Coconut Pecan	1800
White, fluffy	840
All other flavors	2040

GELATIN, ½ cup

Borden's
Cherry	80
Fruit Cocktail	109
Mandarin Orange	89
Perfection	81
Pineapple-papaya	78
Pineapple-raspberry	77
Strawberry	75

Jell-O
1-2-3	81
Best	77

Knox unflavored, dry, 1 envelope   28

Royal   80

JELLIES AND BUTTERS, 1 Tbsp

Apple Butter
Bama	31
Smucker's	
Cider	39
Spiced	39
Peach	45
Ma Brown	32
Musselman's	33

Jams
Ann Page	51
Bama	51
Diet Delight	22
Kraft	49
S & W	10
Smucker's	54
Slenderella	24
artificially sweetened	1

11

Jellies

Ann Page	54
Bama	51
Crosse & Blackwell	51
Diet Delight	21
Home Brands	54
Kraft	48
Low Calorie	22
Ma Brown	49
Musselman's	53
S & W	12
Smucker's	51
Slenderella	24
Single Service	50
Welch's	50

Marmalade

Ann Page	54
Bama	54
Kraft	54
Low Calorie	25
S & W	11
Smucker's	49
Slenderella	24

Preserves

Ann Page	54
Bama	51
Crosse & Blackwell	59
Empress	54
Home Brands	54
Kraft	48

Low Calorie	25
Regular	55
Ma Brown	51
S & W	11
Smucker's	54
Welch's	54
Spreads	
Smucker's	24
Tillie Lewis	12

SPREADS, 1 Tbsp

Anchovy Paste	
Crosse & Blackwell	20
Chicken	
Swanson	35
Underwood	32
Chicken Salad	
Carnation	31
Corned Beef	
Underwood	28
Ham	
Carnation	26
Hormel	35
Libby's	100
Underwood	48

11

Liverwurst
   Underwood   46
Peanut Butter
   Ann Page   105
   Bama   100
    and jelly   82
   Datetree   93
   Home Brands   100
   Jif   93
   Kitchen King   95
   Peter Pan   94
   Planters   95
   Roberts   93
   Skippy   95
   Smucker's   95
    Goober Grape   63
   Sultana   101
Potted Meat
   Libby's   140
Roast Beef
   Underwood   29
Sandwich Spread
   Best Foods   60
   Hellman's   58
   Mrs. Filbert's   53
   Nu Made   51
   Oscar Mayer   33
Spam
   Hormel   40

Tuna
  Carnation   26
Turkey Salad
  Carnation   27

SUGAR, SYRUPS,
SWEETENERS AND HONEY

Honey, 1 Tbsp	64
1 cup	1,031
Sugar, 1 cup	
Brown	
loosely packed	540
firmly packed	820
Maple	790
Powdered	460
sifted	385
White, granulated	770
1 Tbsp	45
Sweeteners, Sugar Substitutes	
Dia-Mel Sugar-Like, 1 gram pkt	3
Dia-Mel Sweet'n-it Liquid	0
Featherweight Sug'r Like, 1 tsp	2
Pillsbury Sprinkle Sweet, 1 tsp	2

Pillsbury Sweet 10	0
Sweet'n Low, 1 gram pkt	3½
Weight Watchers Sweet'ner, 1 gram pkt	3
Whitlock Suprose, 1 gram pkt	4
Syrup, 1 Tbsp	
Aunt Jemima	53
Cary's Diet	10
Cary's Maple	60
Diet Delight	15
Golden Griddle	50
Karo	60
Corn	58
Maple	54
Log Cabin	
Buttered	52
Country Kitchen	53
Maple	46
Maple-Honey	55
Mrs. Butterworth's	54
S & W	12
Tillie Lewis	14
Molasses	
dark	45
light	50
Sorghum	55

CHAPTER 12

Candies, Ice Cream and Nuts

CANDY, 1 oz

Baby Ruth	135
Butterfinger	130
Butter mint	
Kraft	8
Caramel	
Curtiss	113
Kraft	114
Sugar Daddy	113
Sugar Babies	113
Caramel, chocolate-coated	
Kraft	124

Jellied Candy

Dots	100
Jujubes	50
Jujyfruits	94
Mason	99
Quaker City	93
Red Hot Dollars	94

Licorice

Black Crows	101
Diamond Drops	98
Good & Plenty	99
Heide Pastilles	96
Switzer	97

Lifesavers, 1 piece   7

Malted Milk

Walter Johnson	131

Mars   126

Marshmallows

Campfire	100
Curtiss	97
Kraft	96
Jet Puff	125
Macaroon	110

Milky Way   119

Mints

Kraft	105
Richardson	110

Mints, chocolate-coated

Mason	203

12

GUM, 1 piece

Adams	9
Beeman	10
Beech-Nut	9
Beechies	6
Black Jack	9
Bubble Yum	25
Bubblicious	24
Care Free	8
Chiclets	6
Clorets	6
Clove	5
Dentyne	5
Estee	3
Freshen-Up	9
Fruit Stripe	9
Orbit	8
Trident	5
Wrigley's	10

ICE CREAM, 1 cup (½ pint)

Black Raspberry
Breyer's — 264
Black Walnut
Meadow Gold — 329
Butter Almond
Sealtest — 326
Butter Almond and Chocolate
Breyer's — 318
Butter Brickle
Sealtest — 299
Butter Pecan
Meadow Gold — 300
Sealtest — 322
Butterscotch Pecan
Breyer's — 302
Caramel Pecan
Breyer's — 320
Cherry
Sealtest — 276
Cherry-Vanilla
Breyer's — 280
Meadow Gold — 280
Sealtest — 265
Chocolate
Borden's — 255
Breyer's — 314

Carnation	253
Howard Johnson's	519
Meadow Gold	278
Sealtest	281
Swift's	257
Chocolate Almond	
Breyer's	366
Dutch	299
Sealtest	324
Chocolate Chip	
Breyer's Mint	344
Meadow Gold	295
Sealtest	291
Coconut	
Sealtest	321
Coffee	
Breyer's	287
Sealtest	288
Lemon	
Sealtest	272
Maple Walnut	
Sealtest	322
Peach	
Meadow Gold	259
Sealtest	253
Pineapple	
Sealtest	251
Strawberry	
Bordens	253
Breyer's	253

Howard Johnson's	414
Meadow Gold	281
Sealtest	254
Swift's	242
Vanilla	
Bordens	246
Breyer's	299
Carnation	250
Howard Johnson's	500
Meadow Gold	280
Sealtest	289
Swift's	267
Sealtest	280
Vanilla-Fudge	
Breyer's	300
Vanilla-Raspberry	
Sealtest	279

Ice Milk, 1 cup   200

Sherbet, 1 cup   260

Ice Cream Bars, 1

Bi-sicle	110
Creamsicle	78
Dreamsicle	70
Dreamstick	180
Drumstick	183
Fudgesicle	100
Good Humor	
Almond	218
Chocolate	222
Ice	50
Chocolate-covered vanilla	169
Whammy	105
Popsicle	72
Sealtest	
Orange Cream	71
Orange Treat	89

Ice Cream Cones and Cups, 1 item

Comet	
cone	19
cone, rolled sugar	35
cup	20

12
Take-Out Ice Cream, 1 item

Baskin Robbins
Banana Daiquiri Ice	129
Butter Pecan	195
Chocolate Fudge	229
Chocolate Mint	189
Jamoca	182
Mango Sherbert	132
Peach	165
Rocky Road	205
Strawberry	168
Vanilla	217

Bridgeman's
Plain cone	170
Sugar cone	200

Dairy Queen
Banana Split	540
Cone	
large	340
medium	230
small	110
Float	330
Freeze	520
Malt	
large	840
medium	600
small	340
Parfait	460
Sandwich	140

Sundae	
large	400
medium	300
small	170
Friendly's	
Fribble	
chocolate	470
vanilla	420
Sundae	
vanilla fudge	420
vanilla strawberry	340

NUTS AND SEEDS, 1 oz

Almonds	
Blue Diamond	179
Franklin	154
Granny Goose	155
Planters	170
Cashews	
A & P	170
Frito-Lay	170
Franklin	145
Granny Goose	170
Planters	170
Skippy	163

Filberts
Franklin   164

Mixed
A & P   190
Excel   190
Franklin   160
    with peanuts   156
Granny Goose   168
Planters   180
    with peanuts   185
Skippy   172

Peanuts
A & P   180
    in shell   170
Excel   180
Frito-Lay   175
    in shell   160
    Spanish   170
Granny Goose   168
Planters   170
    Spanish, dry roasted   162
    Peanut Crisps   150
Skippy   165
Tavern Nuts   171

Pecans
A & P   200
Granny Goose   203
Planters   190

Pistachios
Frito-Lay   174

Granny Goose	176
Planters	169
Sesame Mix	
Planters	163
Soybeans	
Malt-O-Meal	
dry roasted	132
oil roasted	141
Planters	133
Sunflower Seeds	
whole, 1 lb	1,371
whole, 1 cup	257
hulled, 1 cup	810

CHAPTER 13

Fast Foods and Snacks

CHIPS, PUFFS, CRISPS, ETC.
1 oz unless noted

13

13

Salted	121
Sesame	119
Whole wheat	122

Taco Chips
Old London 127

Tortilla Chips
Doritos
Nachos	137
Tacos	142

Granny Goose 144
Planters
Nachos	128
Tacos	132

Wheat Chips
Bakon Snacks 147

PIZZA, FROZEN, 1 whole
pizza unless noted

Beef and Cheese
El Chico
with enchilada	1,010
with taco	990

Bacon
Tostino's 704

Cheese
Buitoni — 276
Celeste — 473
  large — 1,280
  Sicilian — 1,395
  with mushroom, small — 459
  with mushroom, large — 1,205
Chef Boy-Ar-Dee — 798
  small — 160
Jeno's — 840
  Deluxe — 1,470
  Junior — 165
  Mix — 838
Kraft — 822
  Pee Wee — 170
Lambrecht — 909
La Pizzeria — 1,230
Lean Cuisine — 170
Roman — 891
Stouffer's — 330
Tostino's — 882

Cheese and Refried Beans
El Chico — 902

Cheese and Chili
El Chico — 1,039

Combinations
Celeste — 600
  large — 1,480
Jeno's Deluxe — 1,667

La Pizzeria	830
large	1,529
Stouffer's	789
Tostino's	1,683
Classic	1,675
Hamburger	
Jeno's	888
Tostino's	910
Crisp	955
Open Face	
Buitoni	250
Pepperoni	
Celeste	540
large	1,438
Chef Boy-Ar-Dee	175
Jeno's	901
La Pizzeria	1,322
Roman	889
Stouffer's	800
Tostino's	923
Crisp	960
Classic	1,792
Classic with mushrooms	1,497
Rolls	
Jeno's	
Cheeseburger	268
Pepperoni	262
Sausage	259
Shrimp	214

Sausage

Celeste	561
large	1,500
Jeno's	899
Deluxe	1,495
Mix	1,058
Kraft	1,000
Pee Wee	190
Lambrecht	1,005
La Pizzeria	860
large	1,515
Roman	233
Tostino's	938
Crisp	981
Classic	1,799

POPCORN AND PRETZELS

Popcorn, 1 cup

Jiffy Pop	31
Jolly Time	31
King Korn	
Cheese	40
Seasoned	42
Pops-Rite	38

Presto-Pop	37
3 Minute	38
TNT	52
Wise	43
Cheese-flavored	49
Wonder	45
Pretzels, 1 piece	
Bachman	
B's	8
Beer	55
Medium	20
Teeny	11
Thin	18
Old London	5
Nabisco Mister Salty	
Dutch	51
3-Ring	12
Veri-Thin	20
Pretzelettes	6
Sunshine	19

FAST FOODS

Arby's	
Beef and Cheese Sandwich	450
Club Sandwich	560

Ham and Cheese Sandwich	380
Junior Roast Beef Sandwich	220
Roast Beef Sandwich	350
Super Roast Beef Sandwich	620
Swiss King Sandwich	660
Turkey Deluxe Sandwich	510
Turkey Sandwich	410

Arthur Treacher's

Chicken	271
Chicken Sandwich	265
Chips	243
Chowder	66
Cole Slaw	144
Fish	241
Fish Sandwich	282
Krunch Pup	358
Lemon Luvs	324
Shrimp	380

Brazier (Dairy Queen)

Hamburger	260
Cheeseburger	320
Big Brazier	460
Big Brazier with Cheese	550
Big Brazier with Lettuce and Tomato	470
Super Brazier (The Half-Pounder)	780
Hot Dog	270
Hot Dog with Chili	330
Hot Dog with Cheese	330
Fish Sandwich	400
Fish Sandwich with Cheese	440

French Fries	200
French Fries, large	320
Onion Rings	300

Burger Chef

Chocolate Shake	310
Big Chef	542
Cheeseburger	304
Double Cheeseburger	434
Double Hamburger	325
French Fries	187
Hamburger	258
Mariner Platter	680
Rancher Platter	640
Shake	326
Skipper's Treat	604
Super Chef	600

Burger King

Whopper	650
Double Beef *Whopper*	850
Whopper with Cheese	760
Double Beef *Whopper* with Cheese	970
Whopper Junior	360
Whopper Junior with Cheese	420
Whopper Junior with Double Meat	490
Whopper Junior Double Meat with Cheese	550
Hamburger	310
Hamburger with Cheese	360
Double Meat Hamburger	440
Double Meat Hamburger with Cheese	540

Steak Sandwich	600
Whaler	660
Whaler with Cheese	770
Onion Rings, large	330
Onion Rings, regular	230
French Fries, large bag	360
French Fries, regular bag	240
Chocolate Milkshake	380
Vanilla Milkshake	360
Apple Pie	240

Carl's Jr.

Famous Star Hamburger	480
Super Star Hamburger	660
Old Time Star Hamburger	440
Happy Star Hamburger	290
Steak Sandwich	630
California Roast Beef Sandwich	380
Fish Fillet Sandwich	550
Original Hot Dog	340
Chili Dog	360
Chili Cheese Dog	400
American Cheese	40
Salad with Condiments 11 oz	170
Dressing, 2 oz	
Blue Cheese	200
Thousand Island	190
Lo-Cal Italian	48
French Fries	220
Apple Turnover	330

Carrot Cake	380
Shake	310
Soft Drinks	200
***Church's Fried Chicken*, 1 piece, boned**	
Dark	305
White	327
Dunkin' Donuts	
Cake and Chocolate Cake Donuts	
rings, sticks, crullers, etc.	240
Yeast-raised Donuts	160
Glazed Yeast-Raised Donuts	168
Fancies	
coffee rolls, danish, etc.	215
Fancies with Filling and Topping	260
Munchkins, Yeast-raised	26
Munchkins, Cake and Chocolate Cake	66
Munchkins with Filling and Topping	79
Gino's	
Apple Pie	238
Cheeseburger	300
Cheese Hero	738
Cheese Sirloiner	532
Coke	117
Fish Platter	650
Fish Sandwich	450
French Fries	156
Giant	569
Hamburger	254
Hero	647
Hot Chocolate	90

Hardees

Apple Turnover	282
Big Twin	447
Cheeseburger	335
Deluxe	675
Double Cheeseburger	495
Fish Sandwich	468
French Fries, large	381
French Fries, small	239
Hamburger	305
Hot Dog	346
Milkshake	391
Roast Beef Sandwich	390

Jack-in-the-Box

Apple Turnover	411
Breakfast Jack	301
Cheeseburger	
Deluxe	310
Jumbo Jack	628
Double Cheese Omelet	423
French Fries	270
French Toast	537
Hamburger	
Bonus Jack	461
Deluxe	260
Jumbo Jack	551
Ham and Cheese Omelet	425
Jack Burrito	448
Jack Steak	428
Lemon Turnover	446

Moby Jack	455
Onion Rings	351
Pancakes	626
Ranchero Omelet	414
Scrambled Eggs	719
Shakes, Chocolate	365
Strawberry	380
Vanilla	342
Taco	189
Taco Super	285

Kentucky Fried Chicken

Chicken Dinner
(3 pieces chicken, potatoes, cole slaw, roll)

Original Recipe Dinner	830
Extra Crispy Dinner	950

Individual Pieces

Wing	151
Drumstick	136
Keel	253
Rib	242
Thigh	276

Long John Silver's

Breaded Clams	465
Breaded Oysters	460
Chicken planks	458
Cole Slaw	138
Corn on the Cob	174
Fish with Batter, 2 pieces	318
Fries	375

Hush Puppies	153
Ocean Scallops	257
Peg Leg	514
Shrimp	268
Treasure Chest	467

McDonald's

Apple Pie	300
Big Mac	541
Cheeseburger	306
Cherry Pie	298
Chocolate Shake	364
Egg McMuffin	352
English Muffin, Buttered	186
Fillet O' Fish	402
French Fries	211
Hamburger	257
Hot Cakes, with Butter or Syrup	472
McDonaldland Cookies	294
Quarter-pounder	418
Quarter-pounder with Cheese	518
Sausage	184
Scrambled eggs	162
Shake, Strawberry	345
Shake, Vanilla	323

Pizza Hut, 1 slice, Thin

Standard

Cheese	180
Pepperoni	202
Pork and Mushroom	196

Super Supreme	266
Superstyle	
Cheese	213
Pepperoni	233
Pork and Mushroom	230
Supreme	216
Ponderosa, **Entree**	
Chopped Beef	324
Double Deluxe	362
Extra-cut Prime Rib	409
Extra-cut Ribeye	358
Fillet of Sole	251
Fillet of Sole Sandwich	125
Junior Patty	98
Prime Rib	286
Ribeye	259
Ribeye/Shrimp	400
Shrimp	220
Steakhouse Deluxe	181
Strip Sirloin	277
Super Sirloin	383
T-Bone	374
Poppin' Fresh	
Chef's Salad	800
Custard Pie, 1 slice	380
Dairy Salad	650
Dinner Salad	250
Doughboy Salad	530
Pumpkin Pie, 1 slice	390

Shrimp Salad	640
Tuna Salad	640

Steak 'N Shake

Steakburger	276
Steakburger with Cheese	352
Super Steakburger	375
Super Steakburger with Cheese	451
Triple Steakburger	474
Triple Steakburger with Cheese	625
Low Calorie Platter	293
Baked Ham Sandwich	451
Toasted Cheese Sandwich	250
Ham & Egg Sandwich	434
Egg Sandwich	275
French Fries	211
Chili and Oyster Crackers	337
Chili	402
Baked Beans	173
Lettuce and Tomato Salad with 1 oz Thousand Island Dressing	168
Chef Salad	313
Cottage Cheese	93
Apple Danish	391
Sundaes	
Strawberry	329
Hot Fudge Nut	530
Brownie Fudge	645
Apple Pie	407
Cherry Pie	334

Cheesecake	368
Brownie	259

Taco Bell

Bean Burrito	343
Beef Burrito	466
Beefy Tostada	291
Bellbeefer	221
Bellbeefer with Cheese	278
Burrito Supreme	457
Combination Burrito	404
Enchirito	454
Pintos Cheese	168
Taco	186
Tostada	179

Wendy's

Cheeseburger	
Single cheese	580
Double cheese	800
Triple cheese	1,040
Chili	230
French Fries	330
Frosty	390
Hamburger	
Single	470
Double	670
Triple	850

White Castle

Cheeseburger	185
Fish	192

13

CHAPTER 14

Home Cooked, Restaurant and Frozen

HOME COOKED AND RESTAURANT DISHES,
1 average portion unless noted

Ambrosia	126
Ambrosia salad	542
Anchovy butter, 1 Tbsp	127
Angel Food Cake	120
Apples, baked	225
Apples, stuffed	265
Apple Brown Betty	547
Apples, candied	355
Apple Caramel	488
Apple cinnamon rings	180
Apple curried rings	155
Apple fried rings	165
Apple, pickled, 1 apple	50
Applesauce	225
Apple turnovers	400
Apricot, Brown Betty	498
Armenian style mussels, stuffed with rice, currants and piñon nuts	528
Arroz con Pollo	655
Artichoke, boiled	146
Artichoke hearts, marinated	75
Artichokes, Jerusalem boiled	163
Artichoke moutarde	374
Artichoke, Provencal-style, braised	127
Artichoke vinaigrette	446
Asparagus, buttered	90
Asparagus, Chinese-style	150
Asparagus Divan, 4 spears	375
Asparagus vinaigrette	170

Aspic	25
tomato	60
Athenian-style braised lamb shoulder	589
Austrian-style cabbage	210
Avgolemono sauce, 1 Tbsp	10
Avocado salad dressing, 1 Tbsp	63
Avocado salad, with Belgian endive	245
with tomato	288
farci, ½	400
de crabe, ½	410
de crevettes, ½	489
mousse	137
vinaigrette, ½	380
Baba Ghanouj, ½ cup	185
Bagel and lox with cream cheese	374
Bahamian style coffee	216
Bahamian style conch chowder	340
Baked Alaska	485
Baklava	350
Banana, baked	200
Banana, flambée	438
Banana tea bread	105
Bannock	119
Barbecued spareribs	500
Barley and mushroom casserole	300
Bavarian Cream	212
Bear, pot roasted	500
Béarnaise sauce, 1 Tbsp	48
Bechamel sauce, 1 Tbsp	36

Beef and Asparagus	929
and Bean Curd	682
and Bean Sprouts	646
and Broccoli	585
Congee	896
Consommé, 1 cup	33
Fondue Bourguignonne	479
and Green Pepper	444
Lo Mein	1,042
and Mushrooms	435
and Noodles in Brown Bean Sauce	685
and Oyster Sauce	689
with Pea Pods and Water Chestnuts	648
and Mushroom Pirog	720
Picadillo	400
Beef Brisket	530
Beef Heart, stuffed	475
Beef Kidneys, braised	275
Beef Roasts	
Pot-au-feu	555
Pot Roast	600
Pot Roast, French-style	715
Pot Roast, German-style	650
Sauerbraten	569
Yankee Pot Roast	746
Beef Short Ribs	485
Beef Steak	
Bracioulini	423
Chicken-fried	935
Chinese-style	345

14

Beets

harvard in sour cream	170
in horseradish	120
pickled, 1 beet	10
Beignet d 'Aubergines, 4 oz	200
Beurre Manié, 1 Tbsp	98
Bhendi Bhaji	85
Bernaise Sauce, 1 Tbsp	46
Billi-Bi	222
Biscuit Tortoni	284
Biscuit, Baking Powder, 1 piece	83
Black Bean dip, 1 Tbsp	36
Black-eyed peas, Southern-style	550
Black forest cake	758
Blancmange	162
Blanquette de Veau	699
Blini, 1 piece	87
with butter	184
with caviar	204
Blintzes, cheese, 1 piece	177
Blood Sausage, 6 oz	708
Blueberry muffins	133
Blueberry waffles	259
Bocconcini	524
Bordelaise sauce, 1 Tbsp	23
Borscht	400
Boston Baked beans	534
Boston Brown Bread, 1 slice	86
Bougatsa, 1 piece	401
Bouillabaisse	600

14

Bourek, 1 piece	98
Brains with Almonds	653
braised	338
with sherry	570
Brandied Peaches, 1 peach	65
Bratwurst, grilled, 6 oz	500
Bratwurst, sauteed, 6 oz	563
Brandy Alexander pie	680
Brandy sauce, 1 Tbsp	44
hard, 1 Tbsp	115
Brandy snaps, 1 piece	98
Brazilian Black Beans	376
Bread sauce, 1 Tbsp	18
Brioche	201
Broccoli amandine	279
Broccoli with Parmesan	105
Brownie, 1 piece	160
Buche de Noel	684
Buffalo Steak, broiled	400
Bulgar, pilaf	290
plain	277
Buttermilk Biscuits, 1 piece	88
Buttermilk salad dressing, 1 Tbsp	9
Butterscotch Brownie, 1 piece	156
Butterscotch Sauce, 1 Tbsp	71
Burrito with Beans	321
with Chili	251
with Beef and Beans	335
Bytky	631

Cabbage

Austrian	227
Baked	106
Colcannon	144
Creole	133
Flemish Red, with Apples	268
Pennsylvania Dutch	155
Pickled, 1 cup	200
Polish	400
Rolls Stuffed with Lamb	372
Sweet and Sour	150
Cacciucco	414
Cacik	100
Caesar salad	299

Cake

Applesauce	205
Cheesecake	424
Cheesecake, Italian style	520
Chocolate	230
Cinnamon and Coffee	135
Coconut cream	240
Devil's food	240
Lemon Chiffon	300
Light Fruit	266
Genoese	120
Marble	195
Petits fours, 1 piece	251
Pineapple Upside-down	255
Rainbow	210
Sachertorte	362

Spice	205
Sponge	100
Wedding	150
Trifle	585
Calamari, Baked	286
Calf's Liver	
sauteed	260
with Bacon	375
with Onions	310
alla Veneziana	310
Cannelloni with Beef	398
with Ricotta	356
with Spinach	397
Cannoli	190
Cantonese fried fish, 4 oz	449
Cantonese Lobster	400
Cantonese Shrimp and Vegetables	372
Capicola, 1 slice	108
Caponata, 1 Tbsp	18
Caramel popcorn ball, 1 piece	212
Carp, Sweet and Sour	332
in Brown Sauce	726
Caviar, 1 oz	89
Carrots with dill, 1 cup	55
Carrot tzimmes	707
Cassoulet	1,000
Catalan beef	776
Cauliflower au gratin	323
Cauliflower salad	180
Caviar au gratin, 2 oz	259

14

Celeri Rémoulade, 4 oz	303
Celeriac, creamed	213
Ceviche	308
Champ	157
Champignon farci gratinée, 1 piece	135
Chantilly Sauce, 1 Tbsp	75
Chard, pureed	107
Char shu ding	300
Charlotte Russe	458
Chasseur Sauce, 1 Tbsp	31
Cheese Boreks	138
Cheese Dumplings, 1 piece	95
Cheese Fondue	1,000
Cheese straws, 10 pieces	283
Cheese sauce, 1 Tbsp	38
Cheese souffle	327
Cherries Jubilee	200

Chestnuts
creamed	400
pureed	327
roasted, 6 oz	245

Chicken
and Almonds	750
and Asparagus	510
Barbecued with Skin and Bones	405
Bhuna	219
and Black Bean Sauce	748
Burmese, in Peanut and Coconut Sauce	845
Cacciatore	468
and Cashews	750

Chop Suey	355
Chow Mein	260
Circassian	950
Crispy Fried, Chinese-style	669
Coq au Vin Blanc	385
Coq au Vin Rouge	408
Creamed	426
Croquettes	440
Dahi	220
Dhan Sak	239
Diavolo	290
Divan	378
Drunken Chicken, Chinese	593
Foo Yong	434
Fricassee	469
Francese	320
Jade	666
Jaipur	795
Jambalaya	533
Kiev	520
a la King	390
Kung Pow	482
Lemon	796
Livers, sauteed	120
Lo Mein	728
Maglai	236
Magyar	457
Marengo	366
Moo Goo Gai Pan	248
Molé	562

Musallam	227
with Mushrooms	528
Pancake, Chinese-style	899
Parmigiana	510
Pizziola	290
Roumanian-style, with Apricots	468
Salad	423
with Snow peas	520
Stew	560
stuffed with rice and mushrooms	362
Sub Gum	638
Sweet and Sour	1,150
Tandoori	366
Teriyaki	878
Tetrazzini	878
Chinese-style, with vegetables	670
Velvet	742
Vino bianco	300
with walnuts	929
Yakitori	253
Zingara	500
and tomato salad	199
Chili	448
Chiles con Queso	327
Chiles Rellenos	442
Chiles de Frijoles	544
Chimichango	288
Chinese style	
Beef	343
Cabbage, quickfried	200

Cabbage, steamed 85
Cabbage, Sweet and Sour 200
Carp, Sweet and Sour 300
Mustard Sauce, 1 Tbsp 5
Egg roll 145
Fried eggs and Rice 324
Fried puffs, 1 piece 86
Fried rice 301
Pork with rice 277
Shrimp with ginger 274
Snow peas 115
Spareribs 565
Sweet and sour sauce, 1 Tbsp 15
Cucumber and soy sauce 62

Chocolate
Chiffon Cake, 1 slice 318
Chip Cookie, 1 piece 75
Eclairs 282
Mousse 316
Profiteroles, 1 piece 153
Sauce, 1 Tbsp 86
Hot Soufflé 339

Chinese fried puffs, 1 piece 86

Chopped Chicken liver, ½ cup 262

Chorizos, 1 link 147

Chutney, 1 Tbsp
Coconut 17
Green Tomato 25
Mango 63

Mint	10
Tomato	30
Clams	
Bisque	200
in Black Bean Sauce, Chinese-style, 1	39
Casino, 1 dozen	536
New England Pie	325
Origanata, 1 dozen	440
Red Sauce	301
White Sauce	142
Cockaleekie	95
Cocoa	175
Coconut Macaroon, 1 piece	57
Cod Kedgeree	333
Coleslaw and caraway salad	238
Court Bouillon	4
Couscous, Boiled	305
Beef	567
Chicken	653
Lamb	600
Coquilles Saint-Jacques	475
Cornbread, 1 slice	100
Corn Fritters	249
relish, 1 Tbsp	16
sticks, per stick	100
Corned beef and cabbage	600
Corned beef hash	400
Coulibiac	288
Crab	
Cakes, Maryland-style	257

Cocktail, ½ cup	92
Deviled	398
Legs, Alaska King	297
Louis	767
Meunière, 2	278
Mornay	513
Newburg Imperial	426
Cranberry Nut Bread, 1 slice	136
Cranberry Relish, 1 Tbsp	44
Cranberry sauce, 1 Tbsp	28
Cream Cheese Dip, with Bacon and Horseradish, 1 Tbsp	74
Cream Puff, 1 piece	251
Creme brulee	655
Creme Caramel	280
Crepes, au champignon, 1 piece	178
Crepes, au jambon gratinée, 1 piece	156
Crepes Suzette, 1 piece	208
Crispy Bass, Chinese-style	484
Croissant, 1 piece	90
Croque Madame	710
Croque Monsieur	710
Croquettes de crevette	263
Croquettes de volaille	493
Cucumber and yogurt sauce, 1 Tbsp	5
Crumpet, 1 piece	80
Cumberland sauce, 1 Tbsp	40
Curried	
Beef	415
Beef Triangles, 1 piece	154

Crispy, Chinese style, 4 oz	820
Eight precious, 4 oz	905
with Orange sauce	490
Peking, 4 oz	835
Pressed, 4 oz	399
Wild roast	256
Szechuan, 4 oz	1,000
Tangerine peel, Chinese-style	782
Dumplings, Chinese-style, 1 piece	95
Dumplings, Peking fried, 1 piece	76
Duxelles sauce, 1 Tbsp	19
East Indian Lentils and Rice	264
Eclairs, 1 piece	285
Eel, jellied	605
Eel and egg pie	623
Eggs	
in Aspic, 1	130
Benedict, 1	286
Custard, steamed Chinese-style	226
Deviled, 1	148
Florentine, 1	165
Foo Yong, 1 foo	322
Fried rice, 1 cup	335
Huevos rancheros, 1	177
Salad	403
Scotch, 1	498
Eggnog, nonalcoholic	243
Eggplant	
Basque-style with peppers and tomatoes	155
Dip, 1 Tbsp	45

Fried	281
Greek-style	195
Greek-style, stuffed	180
Ismir	246
Parmigiana	598
Pisto	135
Ratatouille	510
Stuffed with mushrooms and chickpeas	228
Stuffed with pilaf and raisins	188
Turkish	327
Egg Rolls, Chinese, 1 piece	145
Empanada, with beef	244
Empanada, with chicken	220
Enchilada	
Beef	299
Cheese	270
Chicken	330
Chorizo	267
Escalopes de veau cordon bleu	680
Escargot de bourgogne, 6 pieces	418
Escarole, sautéed	74
Esterhazy steak	994
Falafel	263
Fennel, braised	116
Fettuccine Alfredo	1,550
Fettuccine con Baccala	653
Figs, fresh stewed	195
Finnan Haddie	257
Fish balls, Chinese-style, 8 oz	319

Fish, Jade Chinese-style, 6 oz	547
Lemon Chinese-style, 8 oz	754
Fish mousse	286
Fish piquant en papillote	199
Fish soufflé	300
Flan	263
Flemish red cabbage and apples	248
Floating island	257
Florentines, 1 piece	118
Flounder fillet in black bean sauce	600
Fondue de Gruyère	478
Fragrant noodles with shrimp, Chinese-style	810
Franks in blankets, 1 piece	46
French-fried onion rings	165
French-fried potatoes	227
Frijoles fritos	325
Frijoles Mexicanos	194
Frikadeller	384
Fruit cake, light, 1 slice	264
Fudge, chocolate, 1 piece	78
Fudge Sauce, hot, 1 Tbsp	100
Garlic bread, 1 slice	88
Garlic sauce, 1 Tbsp	11
Gefilte fish	183
Giblet gravy, 1 Tbsp	16
Gingersnaps, 1 piece	97
Gingerbread, 1 slice	206
Gingerbread boys, 1 boy	132
Gnocchi, Cheese	410

Farina parmigiana	385
Potato	314
Goose, Braised with chestnuts and onions	525
German style stuffed with potatoes	488
Roasted with apples and sauerkraut stuffing	842
Goulash	394
Grand Marnier soufflé	262
Grand Marnier with strawberries	110
Granite, 1 cup	263
Grasshopper pie	680
Gravy, 1 Tbsp	
au jus	4
giblet	15
mushroom	22
Greek Salad	235
Greek Gyro	246
Green Olives, 2 large	20
Green Beans with garlic, Chinese-style	205
Green Goddess dressing, 1 Tbsp	89
Grenouilles a l'Anglaise	385
Meuniere	485
Provencale	423
Green pepper, Stuffed	190
with beef and kidney beans	356
Mexican-style	444
Green sauce, 1 Tbsp	82
Grits	150
Guacamole, 1 Tbsp	28
Gumbo, corn	172

Gumbo, shrimp	308
Haddock, Baked	300
Creamy smoked and potato casserole	425
Ham	
in aspic	600
fried with red eye gravy	400
loaf	427
Tetrazzini	590
Hamburger	
bacon	400
broiled	280
cheese	370
chili	285
Pizza	285
mushroom	270
Hash	310
Hawaiian spareribs	409
Herb Butter, 1 Tbsp	125
Herring	
and beets a la Russe	591
in dill sauce	188
in mustard sauce	150
in oatmeal	370
Pickled	217
Rollmops	239
Scandanavian salad	379
in sour cream	127
Hoagie, 1 roll	400
Hog Jowl and Black-Eyed Peas	351
Hollandaise sauce, 1 Tbsp	48

Horseradish cream sauce, 1 Tbsp	77
Horseradish, fresh, 1 Tbsp	5
Hot Chocolate	275
Hot Cross Bun, 1 piece	105
Huevos Rancheros, 1 egg	186
Humus with tahini, ½ cup	364
Hushpuppies, 1 piece	67
Indian Corn Fritters, 1 piece	50
Indian Pudding	371
Indian Rice Pilaf	395
Irish Soda Bread, 1 slice	114
Irish Stew	710
Japanese Salad	
autumn	150
cucumber	48
cucumber and fish	135
cucumber and seaweed	64
lotus root	87
Jelly, homemade, 1 Tbsp	45
Jelly Roll	187
Jhinga Bhajia, 1 piece	37
Jhinga Kari, 10-12 shrimp	609
Jhonnycake, 1 piece	98
Kasha, buckwheat	355
appel-almond	400
Katsudon	829
Kebabs, Indian lamb	231
Kedgeree	318
Keema curry	246
Keftedakia Marinata	410

Keftedes	248
Keftedes Avgolemono	200
Khiri Pachadi	122
Kibbeh	964
Kidneys, braised	289
Kielbasa, fried, 3 oz	350
Kissel	240
Knockwurst, sauteed, 6 oz	538
Korma curry	344
Koulebiaka	1,300
Kourabiedes, 1 piece	75
Kreplach, 1 piece	34
Kugelhupf, 1 slice	187
Ladyfingers, 1 piece	52
Lamb	
braised	490
breast	425
cassoulet	1,050
crown roast	270
dolma	232
kidneys in sour cream	485
riblets, barbecued	840
shanks	372
shish kebab	686
stew	403
Lancashire Hot Pot	552
Lasagne, with cheese	605
with meat	408
with meat balls	1,095
Lebkuchen, 1 piece	84

Leek pie	562
Lemon curd, 1 Tbsp	50
Lemonade	118
Lemon Ice	140
Lemon sauce, 1 Tbsp	28
Lemon Sherbet, 1 cup	290
Lentils, boiled	364
Linguini alla Romana	763
Linzertorte, Viennese, 1 slice	304
Liver, Broiled	280
and onions	306
alla Veneziana	314
Chicken, sautéed	247
Chicken pâté	294
Lo mein pork	333
Lobster	
a l'Americaine	503
Cantonese	393
Fra diavolo	586
Mousse	300
Newburg	483
Thermidor	483
London Broil	389
Lotus Root Cake	70
Louisiana Rice and Kidney Beans	483
Lyonnaise sauce, 1 Tbsp	31
Macaroni, Beef and Tomato Casserole	656
and cheese	482
salad	471
Macaroon, 1 piece	44

Mácedoine of vegetables	155
Madeira wine sauce, 1 Tbsp	29
Madeleines, 1 piece	40
Mandel Torte	523
Mannicotti with cheese	275
Mannicotti with meat	292
Maquereau au vin blanc, 4 oz	192
Marinara sauce, 1 cup	200
Marshmellow cream sauce, 1 Tbsp	49
Marzipan, 1 piece	87
Matzo balls, 1 piece	21
Mayonnaise, 1 Tbsp	130
Meatballs	
Danish	396
hot and spicy	158
Konigsberger klops	573
Savory	399
Swedish	693
Lamb stuffed with bulgar	335
Turkish lamb baked in tomato sauce	556
Meat Loaf, plain	222
Meat Loaf, spicy	621
Melba sauce, 1 Tbsp	34
Meringue, 1 piece	47
Meringue Chantilly, 1 piece	196
Milkshake	569
Mincemeat Pie, brandied	588
Mint sauce, 1 Tbsp	25
Molasses Cookies, 1 piece	58
Molé sauce, 1 Tbsp	24

Moo goo gai pan	244
Mornay sauce, 1 Tbsp	33
Moules	
farcis provencale, 8–10 pieces	324
gratinées Normande, 8–10 pieces	285
Marseille, 8–10 pieces	450
salade de, 8–10 pieces	461
vinaigrette, 8–10 pieces	230
Moussaka	818
Mousse, Avocado	196
Chocolate	306
Fish	282
Mozzarella cheese, breaded and fried	231
Muffin, 1 piece	108
Bran	140
Corn	148
Raisin bran	162
Mushroom gravy, 1 Tbsp	26
Mushrooms	
creamed	200
in madeira	236
marinated	51
sauteed	187
Mushrooms with bamboo shoots	295
Mu shu pork, 2 pancakes	874
Mustard sauce, 1 Tbsp	41
Nachos, 1 piece	40
Nantua sauce, 1 Tbsp	24
Napoleons, 1 piece	402

Napolitos	100
New England boiled dinner	735
Nockerln	163
Noodles in brown bean sauce and pork	891
Noodles in oyster sauce	463
Normandy rock cornish game hen, 1 bird	700
Oatmeal Bread, 1 slice	120
Octopus Mediterranean	350
Okra, fried	175
Omelet	
with caviar, 1 egg	180
Greek, 1 egg	130
Lorraine, 1 egg	167
Lyonnaise, 1 egg	136
with mushroom and tomato, 1 egg	135
Onion frittata, 1 egg	200
Piperade, 1 egg	215
Soufflé, 1 egg	111
Spanish, 1 egg	127
Onion Rings, french-fried	184
Onions, baked, 1 piece	155
Onions, creamed	209
sautéed	150
stuffed	186
Oshi tashi	34
Osso buco	905
Oysters casino, 1 dozen	540
Oysters en Brochette	215
Oysters Rockefeller, 1 dozen	1,000

Oyster Sauce, 1 Tbsp ... 35

Paella
with lobster ... 620
with sausage ... 630
Valenciana ... 548

Pakora (Indian fritters)
Baigon ... 41
Gobhi ... 38
Mixed vegetable ... 54

Pancakes, 1 piece
apple ... 95
blueberry ... 87
buckwheat ... 82
buttermilk ... 73
pecan ... 135
plain ... 85
wholewheat ... 89

Panettone, 1 slice ... 322

Paper-wrapped Chicken, Chinese-style, 1 piece ... 98

Parsley sauce, 1 Tbsp ... 22

Parsnips, roasted ... 211

Pashka ... 300

Pastitsio ... 820

Pâté
de Campagne ... 584
de Canard ... 1,076
de Foie Gras ... 648
de Poisson au Asperges ... 478

Peach
cardinal ... 230

cobbler	500
Melba	354
Peanut brittle, 1 piece	77
Peanut butter cookies, 1 piece	70
Pea pods with water chestnuts	307
Pea pods with mushrooms	261
Pear Helene	602
Peking custard	464
Penuche, 1 piece	41
Pepper, Greek stuffed green	120
Pepper, Greek stuffed with rice	160
Peppermint sauce, 1 Tbsp	46
Pepperoni, 1 slice	26
Pfeffernusse, 1 piece	82
Picadillo	400
Piccalilli, 1 Tbsp	12
Pie	
Apple, country	410
Apple, deep dish	445
Banana Cream	626
Blueberry	475
Boston Cream	265
Chocolate cream	610
Coconut cream	462
Coconut custard	400
Key Lime	693
Lemon Meringue	545
Nesselrode	516
Peach	400
Pecan	585

Barbecued with vegetables, Chinese-style	640
Breaded, Italian-style	423
Choucroute garnie	1,000
with rice, Spanish-style	481
Crown roast	584
Loin, stuffed with apples and prunes	685
Lo mein	849
Red, cooked with chestnuts, Chinese-style	432
Sliced, Chinese-style	306
Sliced with green pepper, Chinese-style	411
Soong	666
Spareribs, barbecued	415
Spareribs, Chinese	555
Stuffed with oysters	400
Subgum chow mein	322
Suckling pig	1,100
Sweet and sour, Chinese-style	643
Sweet and sour stew	629
Szechuan-style with bean curd	576
Tenderloin, roast	345
Twice cooked in brown sauce	625
Twice cooked in Hoisin sauce	548
Teriyaki	453
Portugese Filhos, 1 piece	45
Potato Bread, 1 slice	70
Potatoes	
Anna	186
Au Gratin	310
Dauphine	268
Duchess	209

Subgum, fried, 1 cup	436
Roghan Josh	278
Roquefort dressing, 1 Tbsp	71
Rum Custard	208
Rum sauce, 1 Tbsp	36
Russian dressing, 1 Tbsp	80
Rutabaga, boiled	153
Rye Bread, 1 slice	64
Sachertorte	363
Salad	
Caesar	302
Chef's	413
de Saucisson	410
Green Bean	185
Nicoise	305
Spinach with bacon dressing	147
Tabbouleh	262
Three Bean	310
Waldorf	888
Salami, Italian, 1 slice	87
Salisbury Steak	583
Salmon	
Fume au natural	154
Loaf	230
mousse	312
poached	426
soufflé	335
Salsa, 1 cup	253
Salsa Verde, 1 cup	120
Salsify, creamed	237

Saltimbocca	520
Sandwiches	
Bacon, lettuce, and tomato	268
Bagel with cream cheese	255
Bagel with lox and cream cheese	355
Bologna	355
Cheese, grilled	400
Cheese, grilled with bacon	543
Cheese, grilled with tomato	415
Chopped liver	382
Corned beef	446
Fried egg	225
Lobster salad	255
Meatball with tomato sauce	400
Meatloaf	300
Monte Cristo	920
Pastrami	560
Roast beef, overstuffed	490
Reuben	582
Salami	394
Shrimp salad	250
Steak	353
Tongue, overstuffed	475
Tuna fish salad	324
Turkey club	505
Sangria	93
Sardine Fraiches Marines, 4 oz	328
Sashimi, assorted, 4 oz	100
tako, 4 oz	87
Sate	500

Sauce Supreme, 1 Tbsp	34
Saucisson rémoulade	631
Sauerbraten	570
Sauerkraut, with juniper berries, braised	257
with caraway seeds	72
Sausage and Peppers, 2 pieces	882
Scallops, broiled	210
en Brochette	254
Scampi	178
Scrapple	288
Scungilli marinara	269
Sfogliatelli	244
Shabu-shabu	448
Shepherd's Pie	500
Shish kebab	679
Shortbread, Scottish	152
Shortcake, strawberry	591
Shrimp	
Ajillo, 8 large	466
in almond sauce, 8 large	333
Balls, Chinese-style	286
Batter-fried, Chinese-style, 1 piece	84
with bean curd, 12 medium	980
with black bean sauce, Chinese-style	464
Braised, Chinese-style 12 medium	905
Butterfly, Japanese-style	250
with cashews	536
creole	344
Egg foo yong	356
Fried in shell, Chinese-style, 12 medium	674

Glass	299
in green sauce, Spanish-style 8–10	290
Gumbo	327
Jumbalaya	500
in lobster sauce, Chinese-style, 12 medium	1,250
lo mein	501
with Mexican Chilis, 8–10	401
Newburg	600
One shrimp two flavors, 14 medium	900
Scampi	180
Stir-fried, 12 medium	738
Shu Mai, 1 piece	45
Sweet and sour, 12 medium	1,900
Szechuan pepper	324
Toast, 1 piece	162
Sloppy Joe	318
Snails a la bourguignonne, 1 dozen	320
Snails a la provencale, 1 dozen	300
Sole À L'Américaine	305
Amandine	509
Bonne femme	550
with Crab Sauce	300
Goujons de	460
Meuniere	490
Veronique	600
Sopapilla	128
Sopapilla with honey and cream	209
Soubise sauce, 1 Tbsp	20
Soufflé	
au fromage	197

Clam chowder, New England	283
Chicken noodle	78
Chicken and rice	78
Chicken with bean curd, Japanese-style	74
Consommé	42
Escarole	138
Garlic	197
Gazpacho	192
Hungarian cherry	375
Hungarian cream of barley	204
Minestrone	243
Miso with bean curd	79
Miso with fish balls	142
Mulligatawny	304
Mushroom, cream of	272
Oxtail	329
Pastina	134
Peanut, cream of	520
Potato	209
Pumpkin	150
Sauerkraut	128
Senegalese	314
Stracciatelli	125
Stschy	167
Tortellini	210
Turtle, home style	278
Vegetable, cream of	340
Sour cream and chive, 1 Tbsp	29
Sour Dough Bread, 1 slice	65
Souvlaki	291

Spaghetti, 1 cup

Alfredo	405
Bolognese	357
with butter, cream and parmesan	401
Carbonara	860
Clam sauce, red	300
Clam sauce, white	344
Fagioli	348
with meatballs in sauce	853
Paglia e fieno	506
al pesto	980
Pomodoro	268
with sausage	471

Spatzle	165
Spiedini with anchovy	386
Spinach au gratin	275
Spinach, creamed	144
Spoon bread	632
Spumoni, 1 cup	510
Squid, Mediterranean	390
Stuffed with Rice, Greek-style	354
Squirrel Stew	500
Steamed Chinese sausage	778
Steamed Scallops with cabbage, Chinese-style, 8 pieces	300
Steamed Whole Fish, Chinese-style, 1 lb	902
Stifado	228
Stollen, 1 slice	145
Strawberries Romanoff	322
Strawberry Shortcake	500

Strudel
Almond	398
Apple	360
Cheese	410
Cherry	405
Poppy seed	400

Stuffing, 1 cup
Chestnut and mushroom	472
Corn bread	700
Herbed	210
Rice	263
Sage and onion	220

Submarine, 1 roll	381
Sukiyaki	348

Sushi
Chirashi	460
Norimaki	468
Tekka maki	400

Sweet and Sour Chinese meatballs	936
Sweet and Sour fish, 1 lb	902
Sweet and Sour sauce, 1 Tbsp	20
Tabbouleh	304

Tacos
Bean	275
Cheese	205
Chicken	245
Chili	348
Chorizo	367

Taffy, 1 piece	50
Tahini sauce, ¼ cup	167

14

Tamale pie	268
Tandoori fish	300
Shrimp, 10–12	288
Taramasalata, 1 Tbsp	100
Tartar sauce, 1 Tbsp	92
Tarte au champignon	382
au Oignons	570
Tea Eggs, 1 egg	85
Tempura	590
Tempura sauce, 1 Tbsp	5
Teriyaki	
Beef	213
Chicken	380
Pork	462
Teriyaki sauce, 1 Tbsp	15
Toad in the Hole	700
Toast, French, 1 slice	143
Toll House Cookies, 1 piece	60
Tomato Aspic	73
Tomatos, broiled	126
Tomato sauce, 1 Tbsp	10
Bolognese, 1 cup	330
Italian-style, 1 cup	215
with red clam, 1 cup	300
Tomatos, stewed	43
Tortellini with butter and parmesan	582
with ricotta and cream	600
Tortillas, 1 piece, plain	75
Chili	196
Chorizo	500

Sweetbreads

braised	300
creamed	535
with mushrooms	575
sauteed	200
with sherry	585
Terrine of Veal and Ham	250
Vitello Tonnata	850
a la zingara	602
Venison Burgers	360
Ragout of	437
Roast saddle of	205
Vichyssoise	410
Vinaigrette, 1 Tbsp	100
Weiner Schnitzel	415
a la Holstein	457
White sauce, 1 cup	400
Wild Boar, pot roast	500
Wild Duck, roasted	265
Won ton, fried sweet, 1 piece	59
Yakinasu, 4 oz	38
Yakitori	263
Yakitori donburi	781
Yam, candied	315
Yankee pot roast	775
Yogurt kholodnyk	40
Yogurt sauce, 1 Tbsp	9
Yorkshire Pudding	78
Yorkshire Scones, 1 piece	150
Yudofu	83

Zabaglione	177
Zeppole, 1 piece	42
Zucchini, Fried, 1 strip	37
Italian style	100
Sautéed, ½ cup	71
Zuppa di pesce	458
Zuppa Inglese	378

FROZEN DINNERS,

1 complete dinner (see also pp 141-144 and pp 150-153)

Beans and Franks	
Banquet	591
Morton	530
Swanson	550
Beef	
Banquet	312
Chopped	443
La Choy	342
Lean Cuisine Oriental	280
Morton	270
Chopped	340

Country Table	540
Steak House	920
Swanson	370
3-Course	490
Chopped	460
Hungry Man	540
Hungry Man 18 oz	730
Weight Watchers 10 oz	387
Weight Watchers 16 oz	586

Beef and Beans
Swanson	500

Beef Stroganoff
Stouffer's	390

Chicken
La Choy	354
Morton	240
Swanson boneless	730
Weight Watchers	330

Chicken and Biscuits
Green Giant	200

Chicken Croquettes
Morton	410

Chicken Cacciatore
Stouffer's	313
Weight Watchers	356

Chicken and Dumplings
Banquet	282
Morton	280

Chicken, fried
Banquet	530

Man Pleaser	1,026
Morton	470
Country Table	710
Swanson	570
3-Course	630
Hungry Man	620
Hungry Man, 15¼ oz	910
Hungry Man, Barbecue	760
Crispy Fried	650
Chicken, glazed	
Lean Cuisine	270
Chicken with noodles	
Morton	260
Chicken, oriental	
Weight Watchers	320
Chicken Parmigiana and Spinach	
Weight Watchers	200
Chicken and vegetables	
Lean Cuisine	260
Chop Suey	
Banquet	282
Chow Mein	
Banquet	282
Green Giant	130
Lean Cuisine	240
Enchilada	
Banquet	
Beef	479
Cheese	459
El Chico	680

Swanson	570
Van de Kamp	
Beef	420
Cheese	430
Fish	
Banquet	382
Haddock	419
Perch	434
Lean Cuisine	200
Morton	270
Weight Watchers	
Flounder	240
Haddock	250
Perch	320
Sole	240
Turbot	490
Fish and Chips	
Swanson	450
Hungry Man	760
Ham	
Banquet	369
Morton	440
Swanson	380
Hash	
Banquet	372
Italian	
Banquet	446
Swanson	420
Lasagna	
Lean Cuisine Zucchini Lasagne	260

Lean Line	270
Swanson	740
Macaroni and beef	
Banquet	394
Morton	260
Swanson	400
Macaroni and cheese	
Banquet	326
Morton	320
Swanson	390
Manicotti	
Lean Line	270
Meat Loaf	
Banquet	412
Morton	340
Country Table	480
Swanson	530
Meatball	
Swanson	400
Mexican	
Banquet	571
Combination	571
El Chico	820
Swanson	600
Pepper	
La Choy	349
Polynesian	
Swanson	490
Pork	
Swanson	470

Queso
   El Chico   810
Salisbury Steak
   Banquet   390
   Morton   290
     Country Table   430
   Swanson   790
     3-Course   490
     Hungry Man   870
Saltillo
   El Chico   790
Sausage with veal, 1 link
   Lean Line   90
Stuffed Shells
   Lean Line   260
Shrimp
   La Choy   325
Spaghetti with beef
   Lean Cuisine   280
Spaghetti and meatball
   Banquet   450
   Morton   360
   Swanson   410
     Hungry Man   660
Swiss Steak
   Swanson   350
Tacos, beef
   El Chico   410
Turkey
   Banquet   293

Man Pleaser	620
Morton	350
Country Table	600
Swanson	360
3-Course	520
Hungry Man	740
Weight Watchers	400
Veal Parmigiana	
Banquet	421
Morton	330
⟩ *Swanson*	520
Hungry Man	910
Weight Watchers	230
Western	
Banquet	417
Morton	410
Swanson	460
Hungry Man	890
Ziti, baked	
Lean Line	270

CHAPTER 15

Fingertip Low Calorie Guide

OVER 350 CALORIES

Frozen entrees (at less than 30 calories per ounce)

Banquet Buffet Supper Beef and Noodles, 32 oz	754
Banquet Buffet Supper Beef Stew, 32 oz	700
Banquet Buffet Supper Chicken and Noodles, 32 oz	764
Banquet Buffet Supper Beef sliced with gravy, 32 oz	782
Banquet Buffet Supper Turkey, 32 oz	564
La Choy Chicken	354

Morton Country Table Salisbury Steak, 15 oz   430

Swanson Hungry-Man Turkey, 13¼ oz   380

Weight Watchers Turkey Tetrazzini, 13 oz   380

200-350 CALORIES

Frozen entrees (at less than 30 calories per ounce)

Beef

Banquet, 11 oz   312

Lean Cuisine, 9⅛ oz   280

Morton, 10 oz   270

Chicken

Morton, 10 oz   240

Stouffer's

Chicken a la King, 9½ oz   330

Creamed Chicken, 6½ oz   300

Chicken Divan, 8½ oz   335

Weight Watchers, 15 oz   330

Chicken and Biscuits

Green Giant, 7 oz   200

Chicken Creole

Weight Watchers, 13 oz   250

Chicken and Dumplings

Banquet, 12 oz   282

Morton, 11 oz   280

Chicken with Noodles
  Green Giant, 9 oz   250
  Morton, 10½ oz   260
Chicken Oriental
  Weight Watchers, 16 oz   320
Chicken Parmigiana and Spinach
  Weight Watchers, 9 oz   200
Chicken and Vegetables
  Lean Cuisine, 12¾ oz   260
Chicken White Meat with Peas
  Weight Watchers, 9 oz   270
Chop Suey
  Banquet, 12 oz   282
Chow Mein
  Banquet, 12 oz   282
  Lean Cuisine, 11¼ oz   240
Eggplant Parmigiana
  Weight Watchers, 13 oz   280
Fish
  Lean Cuisine, 9 oz   200
  Morton, 9 oz   270
  Weight Watchers
    Flounder, 16 oz   240
    Haddock, 16 oz   250
    Perch, 16 oz   320
    Sole, 16 oz   240
    Sole with peas, mushrooms and
      lobster sauce, 9½ oz   200
Green Peppers with Beef
  Green Giant, 7 oz   200

15

Lasagne
Lean Line, 10 oz   270

Lasagne, Zucchini
Lean Cuisine, 11 oz   260

Macaroni with Beef
Green Giant, 9 oz   240
Morton, 10 oz   260

Macaroni and Cheese
Banquet, 12 oz   326
Morton, 11 oz   320

Manicotti
Lean Line, 11 oz   270

Salisbury Steak
Banquet, 11 oz   390
Morton, 11 oz   290

Shells, Stuffed
Lean Line, 11 oz   260

Spaghetti with Beef
Lean Cuisine, 11½ oz   280

Turkey
Banquet, 11 oz   293
Swanson Turkey Slices, 8¾ oz   260

Ziti, Baked
Lean Line, 10 oz   270

Ziti with Veal and sauce
Weight Watchers, 13 oz   350

Veal Parmigiana with Zucchini
Weight Watchers, 9½ oz   230

Canned Entrees (at less than 30 calories per ounce)

Pasta, one can
  Ravioli
    Franco-American Beef, 7½ oz   220
  Rotini
    Franco-American, 7½ oz   200
  Macaroni
    Franco-American, 7½ oz   220
  Macaroni and Meatballs
    Franco-American, 7½ oz   220
Meat, one can
  Beef Goulash
    Hormel, 7½ oz   240
  Ham, whole
    Hormel, 6 oz   312
  Tuna, in water, drained
    Chicken of the Sea solid white, 7 oz can   216

Fish, Fresh

Crab, steamed, meat only, 8 oz   211
Haddock, fillets, 8 oz   180
Halibut, fillets, 8 oz   226
Oysters, Pacific and Western, meat only, 8 oz   207

15

Meat

Beef

Chuck
  boneless, lean only, braised, 4 oz — 219
  boneless, lean only, stewed, 4 oz — 243
Flank steak, boneless, all lean, braised, 4 oz — 222
ground, lean with 10% fat, 4 oz — 203
porterhouse steak with 9% bone, lean only,
  broiled, 4 oz without bone — 254
round steak, boneless, lean only, braised or
  broiled, 4 oz — 296
sirloin steak, 7% bone, lean only, broiled,
  4 oz without bone — 235
T-bone, 11% bone, lean only, broiled, 4 oz
  without bone — 253

Ham

fresh, lean only
  baked, without bone and skin, 4 oz — 246
light cured, lean only
  baked, without bone and skin, 4 oz — 328

Lamb

Leg, lean only, roasted, boneless, 4 oz — 211
loin chops, with bone, lean only, broiled,
  4 oz — 213
rib chops, with bone, lean only, broiled,
  4 oz — 239
shoulder, lean only, roasted, boneless, 4 oz — 233

Pork

Picnic, without bone and skin, lean only, baked
or roasted, 4 oz   239

Veal

loin cuts, lean with fat, braised or broiled,
without bone, 4 oz   245
round with rump (roasts and leg cutlets),
lean with fat, braised or broiled, without
bone, 4 oz   245

Poultry

Chicken

roasted, without skin, 4 oz   204
stewed, light meat without skin, 4 oz   207
Turkey, roasted, light meat without skin, 4 oz 200

101-200 CALORIES

Pasta

All pasta, dry, one cup
cooked till tender, (approx)   190
cooked till firm, (approx)   155

Canned, 1 can

Franco-American macaroni and cheese, 7½ oz   184

Franco-American spaghetti with cheese, 7⅜ oz   170

Franco-American spaghetti with cheese
sauce, 7⅜ oz   160

Meat Entrees (at less than 30 calories per ounce)

Frozen

Beef, chipped, creamed
  Banquet, 5 oz   124

Beef, sliced
  Banquet, barbecue sauce, 5 oz   126
  Banquet, with gravy, 5 oz   116
  Green Giant, 5 oz   130

Beef Stew
  Green Giant Boil-in-Bag, 9 oz   160
  Green Giant, with biscuits, 7 oz   190

Veal steaks
  Hormel, 4 oz   130

Meat Entrees, canned (at less than 30 calories per ounce), 1 can

Beef, corned with cabbage
  Hormel, 8 oz   150
Beef stew
  Dinty Moore, 7½ oz   184
  Swanson, 7½ oz   190
Pork, sliced, with gravy
  Morton House, 6¼ oz   190

Poultry entrees

Frozen (at less than 30 calories per ounce)
  Chicken a la King
    Banquet, 5 oz   138
Canned, 1 can
  Chicken stew
    Swanson, 7½ oz   180
  Turkey slices
    Morton House, 6¼ oz   140
  Chicken, fresh
    Broiled, meat only, 4 oz   154

15

Seafood

Clams, canned, drained, 1 can	
Doxsee, 8 oz	112
Doxsee, 12 oz	147
Shrimp marinara, with shells, frozen	
Buitoni, 4 oz	116

Fish, fresh, 4 oz, meat only

Abalone	111
Black Sea Bass	106
Butterfish, gulf	108
Catfish, fresh water	117
Croaker, Atlantic	109
Lake Herring (Cisco)	109
Lobster	109
Mussels	108
Ocean Pearch, Pacific	108
Red or Grey Snapper	106
Sea bass, white	109
Shrimp	103
Sturgeon	107
Tautog (Blackfish)	101

51-100 CALORIES

Miscellaneous

Pabst Extra Light Beer	70
Whipped butter, 1 Tbsp	65
Farina, *Pillsbury*, ⅔ cup	80
Grits, *Quaker* Instant, 1 packet	79
One Egg, raw or boiled	
extra large	94
large	82
medium	72
Canned Spaghetti with meatballs, *Libby's*, 1 cup	84
Canned Spanish rice, *Libby's*, 1 cup	57

Chinese dishes

Chow mein, canned, 1 cup	
La Choy	
beef	72
chicken	68
mushroom	85
pepper	89
shrimp	61
Chow mein, frozen	
Banquet, 1 bag	89

15

La Choy beef, 1 cup	97
La Choy shrimp, 1 cup	73
Pea pods, frozen, 1 package	
La Choy	90
Won Ton, frozen, 1 cup	
La Choy	92

Dairy

Cottage Cheese, low fat, ½ cup	
Borden	90
Breakstone	90
Friendship	100
Lucerne	100
Viva	100
Weight Watchers	90
Milk, 8 ounces	
Buttermilk	
.1% fat *Borden*	88
.2% fat *Sealtest* skim	71
.5% fat *Borden*	90
.8% fat *Golden Nugget*	92
.8% fat *Light 'n Lively*	95
Dry, non-fat milk, reconstituted	81
Skin or low-fat	
no fat *Lucerne*	90
.1% fat *Borden*	81

fortified	81
.1% fat *Sealtest*	79
Yogurt, plain, ½ cup	
Borden Lite-Line lowfat	70
Sealtest Light 'n Lively lowfat	70
***Danny On-A-Stick*, uncoated**	65

Meat, canned

Beef stew	
Libby's, 1 cup	78
Ham, whole	
Wilson's certified boned and rolled, 1 oz	56

Poultry

Chicken stew with dumplings, canned	
Libby's, 1 cup	88
Turkey with gravy, frozen	
Banquet, 5 oz	98
Green Giant, 5 oz	100

15

Seafood, canned

Clams

Snow's, ½ cup	60
Sau-Sea, 4 oz	99

Gefilte Fish

Manischewitz, 3 oz piece	53
Manischewitz whitefish and pike, 3 oz piece	64
Mother's, 4 oz piece	55

Oysters

Bumblebee, ½ cup	86

Shrimp

Bumblebee, 4½ oz can	90

Seafood, fresh, meat only, 4 oz

Clams	92
Cod	88
Crayfish	82
Croaker, white	95
Flounder	89
Ocean Perch, Atlantic	100
Oysters	75
Pickerel	95
Pike	100
Sand Dab	89
Sauger	95
Scallops	92
Sole	90
Squid	95
Tilefish	90

Fruits and Vegetables

Artichokes
  boiled, drained, 1 whole bud   67
Beets
  raw, diced, 1 cup   58
Broccoli
  boiled, drained, 8 oz   59
Carrots
  raw, slices, 1 cup   53
Chayote
  raw, 1 medium squash   56
Cranberries
  fresh, without stems, 1 cup   52
Currants, red or white
  trimmed, 1 cup   55
Dock or Sorrel
  raw with stems, 1 lb   89
Endive, French or Belgian
  trimmed, 1 lb   68
Escarole
  untrimmed, 1 lb   80
Grapefruit
  pink or red, with seeds
    whole, with skin, 1 lb   87
    sections, 1 cup   80
  pink or red, seedless
    whole, with skin, 1 lb   93
    sections, 1 cup   80

white, with seeds
  whole, with skin, 1 lb   84
  sections, 1 cup   82
white, seedless
  whole, with skin, 1 lb   87
  sections, 1 cup   78

Honeydew Melon
  whole, with rinds and seeds, 1 lb   94
  cubed or diced, 1 cup   56

Lettuce
  Iceberg
    whole, 1 lb   56
  Loose Leaf
    whole, 1 lb   52
  Romaine or cos
    whole, 1 lb   52

Pawpaw
  peeled and seeded, 4 oz   96

Papaya
  peeled and seeded, cubed, 1 cup   55

Peaches
  pared, sliced, 1 cup   65

Raspberries
  black, 1 cup   98
  red, 1 cup   70

Strawberries
  whole, 1 cup   55

Watermelon
  whole, with rind, 1 lb   54

20-50 CALORIES

Breads, Buns and Rolls

Bread, 1 slice
Gluten
  Thomas — 32
Protein
  Thomas — 45
Rice Cakes
  Spiral — 36
Wheat
  Thomas — 50
White
  Arnold Melba Thin — 40
  Fresh Horizons — 50
  Pepperidge Farm Very Thin — 40
  Weight Watchers — 35
Buns and Rolls, 1 piece
  Pepperidge Farm Old-Fashioned — 37
  Pepperidge Farm Party — 35
Margarine, 1 Tbsp
  Blue Bonnet Diet — 50
  Fleischmann Diet — 50
  Imitation — 50

15

Candy, 1 piece

Rolo	28

Cheese, 1 oz

Farmer's	
Friendship	38
Ricotta	
Borden	42
Imitation Cream Cheese	
Philadelphia	50
American, grated	
Borden	30

Chinese Dishes

Apple-Cinnamon roll, frozen	
La Choy, 1 piece	38
Bamboo Shoots, canned	
La Choy, 8 oz	23
Bean sprouts, canned	
La Choy, 8 oz	24
Chow Mein, canned, 1 cup	
Chun King	44
La Choy, meatless	47

Egg Rolls, frozen
  La Choy chicken, 1 piece   30
  La Choy lobster, 1 piece   27
Mixed vegetables, canned
  La Choy, 1 cup   35

Cream

Half & Half, 1 Tbsp   20
  Lucerne Real Cream topping, 1 whipped oz   20

Dips, 1 oz

Bean, Jalapeño
  Frito-Lay   36
  Gebhardt   30
  Granny Goose   37
  Lucerne   36
Clam
  Lucerne   34
Gelatin
  Knox gelatin, 1 envelope   28
Gravy
  French's Pork, mix, ½ cup   40

15

Jelly, 1 Tbsp

Apple
  Kraft, Low Calorie   22
  Diet Delight   22
Apricot Pineapple Jam
  Diet Delight   21
Blackberry Apple
  Kraft, low calorie   22
Blackberry Jam
  Diet Delight   21
Grape
  Kraft, Low Calorie   22
  Diet Delight   21
Raspberry Jam
  Diet Delight   21

Meat, 1 oz, canned

Beef
  Corned, canned
    Safeway   35
  Dried
    Swift   42
  Smoked
    Safeway   35
    Safeway spicy   40

Beef roast	
Wilson	33
Ham	
Wilson certified fully cooked	48
Wilson certified *Tender Made*	44
Wilson certified festival ham	48
Pastrami	
Safeway	40
Scrapple	
Oscar Mayer in tube	50
Oscar Mayer Philadelphia style	45

Olives

Green, 10 large	45
Manzanillo Black, 10 large	50

Popcorn, 1 cup

Pops-Rite, popped	38
Wise, cheese-flavored, ready to eat	49

15 Poultry

Safeway smoked chicken, 1 oz	50
Safeway smoked turkey, 1 oz	50

Pudding, ½ cup

D-Zerta
butterscotch	25
chocolate	20
vanilla	30

Salad Dressing, 1 Tbsp

French
Ann Page Low Calorie	25
Kraft Low Calorie	25
Nu Made Low Calorie	20

Italian
Wish-Bone Low Calorie	20

May Lo Naise
Tillie Lewis	25

Russian
Wish-Bone Low Calorie	25

Thousand Island
  Ann Page Low Calorie   25
  Wish-Bone Low Calorie   25
Whipped
  Tillie Lewis   25

Sauces & Spreads

Crosse & Blackwell Anchovy Paste 1 Tbsp   20
Hunt's Tomato Sauce, 4 oz   35
  with mushrooms, 4 oz   40
Open Pit Barbecue, 1 Tbsp   26

Vegetables, canned and frozen

Artichoke Hearts
  Birds Eye, 3 oz   20
Asparagus, 1 cup, canned
  cuts   40
  spears   40
  spears and tips   35
  whole   50
Asparagus, frozen
  Birds Eye, 3.3 oz   25
  Seabrook Farms, ½ cup   23

Beans, green canned, 1 cup
french

Del Monte	40
Green Giant	30
Kounty Kist	40
Libby's	35

whole

Del Monte	35
Green Giant	30
Kounty-Kist	40
Libby's	35
Stokely-Van Camp	40

Beans, green, frozen

Birds Eye, 3.3 oz	25
Kounty Kist, 1 cup	30
Seabrook Farms, 1 cup	42

Beans, wax or yellow, 1 cup

Del Monte	35
Libby's	40
Stokely-Van Camp	45

Broccoli, frozen

Birds Eye 3.3 oz	25
Green Giant, 1 cup	30
Kounty Kist, 1 cup	30
Seabrook Farms, 1 cup	46

Brussels Sprouts, frozen

Birds Eye, 3.3 oz	30
Green Giant, 1 cup	50
Kounty Kist, 1 cup	50

Carrots, canned, 1 cup
  Libby's 40
  S & W 44
Cauliflower, frozen
  Birds Eye 3.3 oz 25
  Green Giant, 1 cup 25
  Kounty Kist, 1 cup 25
Collard Greens
  Birds Eye, 3.3 oz 30
  Seabrook Farms, 1 cup 44
Mixed Vegetables
  Kounty Kist, California, 1 cup 30
Mustard Greens
  Seabrook Farms, ½ cup 21
Sauerkraut, canned, 1 cup 50
Spinach, canned, 1 cup 45
Spinach, frozen, 1 cup 50
Tomatoes, canned
  Hunt's stewed, 4 oz 30
  Libby's whole, 1 cup 45
  S & W whole, 1 cup 42
  Stokely-Van Camp, whole 50
  Townhouse, whole 50
Turnip Greens
  Birds Eye 3.3 oz 20
  Seabrook Farms, ½ cup 22
  Stokely-Van Camp, ½ cup 22

Fruits and Vegetables, fresh, 1 cup unless noted

Asparagus	
cut spears	35
Bamboo shoots	
cuts	41
Bean Sprouts	37
Beans, green or snap	
cuts	34
Beans, wax or yellow	
cuts	30
Beet Greens	26
Cabbage, red or green, chopped	22
Cantelope, cubed	48
Casaba Melon, cubed	45
Cauliflower, flowerets	27
Swiss Chard, leaves only	32
Eggplant, diced	50
Radish, diced	20
Rhubarb, raw diced	20
Summer Squash, diced	35
Tomatos, sliced	40
Turnips, cubed	39

Fruit and Vegetable drinks, 6 oz

Cranberry	
Ocean Spray low calorie	35

Cranberry apple
Ocean Spray cranapple low calorie   30
Sauerkraut
Libby's   20
Tomato
Campbell's   35
Del Monte   35
Heinz   38
Hunt's   43
Libby's   39
S & W   22
Sacramento   35
Stokely-Van Camp   33
Townhouse   35
Welch's   38
Tomato cocktail
Ortega Snap-E-Tom   38
Vegetable cocktail
S & W   21
Townhouse   35
V-8   35

UNDER 20 CALORIES

Beverages

Note: virtually all sodas that are called *low-calorie*, *sugar-free* or *dietetic* contain 2 calories or less.

Bouillon, 1 cube

Beef
Herb-Ox	6
Maggi	6
Wyler's	7
Wyler's Instant	10

Chicken
Herb-Ox	6
Maggi	7
Wyler's	8
Wyler's Instant	6

Onion
Herb-Ox	10
Wyler's	6

Vegetable
Herb-Ox	6
Wyler's	6

Breath Mints, 1 piece

Certs clear	8
Certs pressed	6
Chewels	10
Clorets mints	6
Dentyne dynamints	2
Lifesavers	7
Trident mints	8

Broth, 1 packet

Herb-Ox
Beef	8
Chicken	12
Onion	14
Vegetable	12

Candy, Dietetic

Estee, 1 piece
chocolate covered raisins	6
gum drops	3
hard candies	12
mint candies	4

Cocktail Mix, non-alcoholic, 1 oz

Holland House Bloody Mary	6
Holland House Whiskey Sour	9

Coffee, 1 cup

ground	2
instant	4

15

Condiments, 1 Tbsp

A-1 sauce	12
Catsup	
Del Monte	15
Chili sauce	
Heinz	17
Horseradish	2
Mustard	
French's Brown	15
French's Yellow	16
Grey Poupon Dijon	15
Soy sauce	
La Choy	8
Taco sauce	
Old El Paso	4
Vinegar	1
Worcestershire	10

Cookies, 1 piece

Angel Puffs	
Stella D'Oro Dietetic	17
Arrowroot	
Sunshine	16
Royal Nuggets	
Stella D'Oro	1

Vanilla Snaps
Nabisco   13
Vanilla Wafers
Sunshine   15
Nabisco   18
Zuzu Ginger Snaps
Nabisco   16

Cough Drops   9

Crackers, 1 cracker

Cheez-It
Sunshine   6
Cheeze
Keebler   11
Flings Curls
Nabisco   10
Matzos
Manischewitz Tam Tams   14
Melba Toast
Old London
Garlic   9
Onion   10
Pumpernickel   17
Rye   17
Sesame   10
Wheat   17
White   17

15

Oyster
Keebler	3
Sunshine	3

Ritz
Nabisco	16

Saltines
Keebler Zesta	12
Nabisco Premium	12
Sunshine Krispy	11

Sociables
Nabisco	10

Triangle Thins
Nabisco	8

Wheat Thins
Nabisco	9

Creamers, Non-Dairy, 1 tsp

Coffee-Mate, Carnation, 1 pkt	11
Coffee-Tone	12
Cremora, Pet	11

Gelatin, mix, ½ cup

D-Zerta	8
Royal Sweet As You Please	6

Gravy, ¼ cup, mix

Au Jus
Durkee	8
French's	8
McCormick	4
Schilling	4

Brown
Durkee	15
Durkee with mushrooms	15
Durkee with onions	17
McCormick Lite	10
Weight Watchers	8
with mushrooms	12
with onions	13

Chicken
Durkee home style	18
McCormick Lite	10
Pillsbury home style	15
Schilling Lite	10
Weight Watchers	10

Mushroom
McCormick	19
Schilling	19

Pork
Durkee	18

Mushroom Steak
Dawn Fresh	4

Swiss Steak
Durkee	11

15

Gum, 1 piece

Adams	9
Beeman	10
Beech-Nut	9
Beechies	6
Black Jack	9
Care Free	8
Chiclets	6
Clorets	6
Clove	5
Dentyne	5
Estee	3
Freshen-Up	9
Fruit Stripe	9
Orbit	8
Trident	5
Wrigley's	10

Jelly, 1 tsp

Ann Page, all flavors	18
Diet Delight Strawberry	18
Kraft, all flavors	16
S & W, all flavors	10
Smuckers Slenderella, all flavors	8

Oil

Pam Vegetable spray	7

Pickles

Capers, 1 Tbsp
Crosse & Blackwell	6

Onions, cocktail, 1 Tbsp
Crosse & Blackwell	1

Peppers, 1 oz
Chile Green, *Ortega*	5
Hot Pickled, *Old El Paso*	9

Dill Pickles, spears, 1 piece
Bond's	2
Del Monte	7
Heinz	7
Smucker's	8

Sour Pickles, 1 piece
Del Monte	10

Salad dressings, 1 Tbsp

Blue Cheese
Ann Page Low Calorie	18
Kraft Low Calorie	14

   Tillie Lewis   12

   Weight Watchers   10

Caesar

   Pfeiffer Low Calorie   10

French

   Pfeiffer Low Calorie   18

   Weight Watchers   4

   Tillie Lewis   12

Italian

   Ann Page Low Calorie   14

   Kraft Low Calorie   6

   Nu Made Low Calorie   16

   Pfeiffer Low Calorie   10

   Tillie Lewis   6

   Weight Watchers   2

Red Wine

   Pfeiffer Low Calorie   10

Russian

   Pfeiffer Low Calorie   15

   Tillie Lewis   12

   Weight Watchers   12

Thousand Island

   Pfeiffer Low Calorie   15

   Tillie Lewis   18

   Weight Watchers   12

Sauces, 1 Tbsp

Barbecue
  French's   14
Enchilada
  Old El Paso hot   9
  Old El Paso mild   10
Lemon-Butter
  Weight Watchers   8

Sugar, 1 tsp   15

Pancake Syrup, 1 Tbsp

Cary's **Diet**   10
Diet Delight   15
S & W   12
Tillie Lewis   14

Tea, 1 cup   1

lemon-flavored
  Nestea   2

15

Toppings, 1 Tbsp

No-Cal
  all flavors except chocolate and coffee   0
  No-Cal chocolate & coffee   6
whipped mix
  D-Zerta   8
  Dream Whip   10

Vegetables and Fruits, Fresh

Cabbage
  Chinese, cuts, 1 cup   11
  spoon (Bakchoy), cuts, 1 cup   11
Celery
  1 large outer stalk   7
  3 small inner stalks   9
Chicory greens
  cuts, 1 cup   11
  10 inner leaves   5
Endive, French or Belgian
  1 head, 5-7"   8
  10 small leaves   5
  chopped, 1 cup   14
Escarole, cuts, 1 cup   10
Mushrooms, chopped, 1 cup   20
Pepper, sweet, green, sliced, 1 cup   18

Pickles
  dill, 1 large   15
  sour, 1 large   14
Spinach, trimmed and chopped, 1 cup   14
Watercress, 1 cup   7